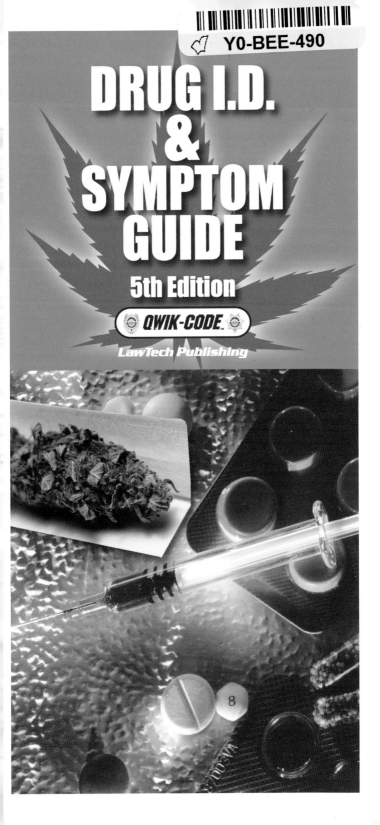

DRUG I.D. & SYMPTOM GUIDE

5th Edition

QWIK-CODE™

LawTech Publishing

Copyright ©2010 *LawTech Publishing Co., Ltd.*

QWIK-CODE is a registered trademark of *LawTech Publishing Co. Ltd.*.

LawTech Publishing
1(800)498.0911
www.LawTechPublishing.com

Comments and suggestions are welcome.
info@LawTechPublishing.com

Special Thanks to:

Trinka Porrata, Contributing Editor - Founder and President, Project GHB, www.projectghb.org

Jim Aumond, Training Director, California Narcotic Officers' Association. www.cnoa.org

Teri Bennett, Supervising Investigator, Medical Board of California, for her photo contributions of Butalbital, Demerol vials, Provigil, OxyContin and Zyprexa.

pp. 224

Printed in China

ISBN: 978-1-56325-166-5

CONTENTS

CANNABIS
Marijuana 2
Marijuana Cigarette/Thai Stick 4
Marijuana Grow 6
Hashish Oil 8
Hashish. 10

DEPRESSANTS
Alcohol (Ethanol) 14
Barbiturates 16
Non-Barbiturates 18
Anti-Psychotic Tranquilizers 20
Benzodiazepines 22
GHB/Xyrem/GBL/BD/Other Analogs 24
Miscellaneous Depressants 28
Anti-Depressants 30

HALLUCINOGENS
Phenethylamines 34
MDMA - Phenethylamines 35
Tryptamines 40
Jimson Weed 44
LSD. 46
Peyote 50
Psilocybin & Psilocin 52
Salvia Divinorum. 54
Nutmeg – Myristicin. 56
Miscellaneous Hallucinogenic Stimulants. 58

INHALANTS
Inhalant Abuse (General) 62
Amyl/Butyl Nitrite
Cyclohexyl Nitrite 66
Nitrous Oxide 68

NARCOTICS
Codeine. 72
Fentanyl 74
Heroin. 76
Cheese 80
Hydromorphone 82
Hydrocodone 84
Meperidine 86
Methadone 88
Morphine 90
Opium. 92
Oxycodone 94
Additional Narcotics 96
Kratom 98

DISSOCIATIVE ANESTHETICS
PCP. 102
Ketamine. 104
Dextromethorphan 106

STIMULANTS
Amphetamines 110
Cocaine. 112
Cocaine. 114
Methamphetamine 116

Methcathinone 118
Cathinone 120
Additional Stimulants 122

ANDROGENIC ANABOLIC STEROIDS **126**

PARAPHERNALIA IDENTIFICATION AND DESCRIPTIONS

Marijuana Smoking Paraphernalia. 130
Marijuana Roach Clips 131
Other Types of Smoking Paraphernalia. 132
Freebase Smoking pipe 133
Methamphetamine (ICE) Smoking Pipes. 134
Bindle 136
Cocaine Sifter 137
Snorting Cocaine 138
Copper Scouring Pads 139
Drug Lab 140
Heroin Paraphernalia. 141
Nitrous Oxide Paraphernalia 142
Rave Paraphernalia. 144
Scales. 146
Snorting Spoon. 147
Snorting Tube 148
Snorting Vials 149
Stash Cans 151
Wash-Back Methods 153
Clothing Indicates Drug Preference. 154
Clothes That Hide Drugs 155

NEEDLE INJECTIONS/ PUNCTURE WOUNDS

Sterile Injections. 160
Unsterile Injections. 160

APPENDIX

Autoerotic Asphyxiation, The Choking Game & Cutting . . 164
Drug-Facilitated Sexual Assaults 165
Drug Statistics 166
Early Warning Signs 169
Gateway Drugs. 170
Drug Evaluation & Testing. 171
Drug Testing 176
Detection Limits 177
Weights & Measures 179
Drug Abuse in the Workplace. 180
Workplace Drug Abuse Resources 181

DEFINITIONS

Definitions 183
Street Slang 184

INDEX. **217**

CANNABIS

MARIJUANA
Cannabis

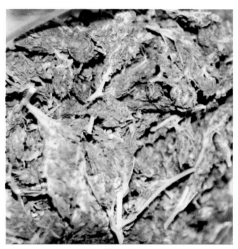

Dried Marijuana

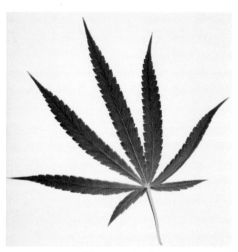

Marijuana Leaf

MARIJUANA
Cannabis

Visual Description:
A dried, green leafy substance mixed with stems and possibly seeds.

Methods of Use:
Ingested, Smoked

Effects:
Onset: 8-10 Seconds
Peak: 10-30 Minutes
Duration: 6-8 Hours

Symptoms of Use:
Nystagmus – No
Pupils – Normal (possibly dilated)
Pulse – Elevated
Blood Pressure – Elevated
Body Temperature – Near normal
Non-Convergence – Yes
Bloodshot eyes
Body tremors
Debris in mouth
Difficulty concentrating
Disoriented
Eyelid tremors
Impaired divided attention
Impaired time/distance perception
Increased appetite
Odor of burning marijuana
Rebound dilation
Relaxed inhibitions

Overdose Symptoms:
Fatigue
Paranoia
Psychosis

Additional Comments:
Foil packets labeled with names like Spice, Spice Gold, Spice Silver, Spice Diamond, Genie and Yucatan Fire "incense" have recently surfaced. While negative by standard marijuana testing, these products were shown to contain a variety of herbs plus verifiable amounts of synthetic cannabinoids or cannabinoid-mimicking compounds, including HU-210 and/or JWH-018. Herbal products Skunk and Sence also tested positive for HU-210, and are reputedly more potent than THC, making even small amounts potentially physiologically active. This is a rapidly emerging abuse issue worldwide, resulting in bans in several European countries in 2009. Legislation regarding these products is on the horizon for the U.S. and some states have initiated legislation. This drug combination is also known as K2.

MARIJUANA CIGARETTE/THAI STICK

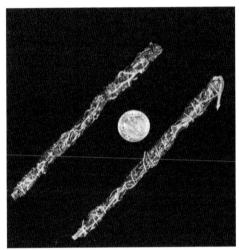

Thai Sticks

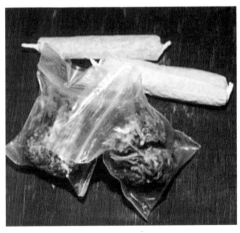

Packaged Marijuana and Marijuana Cigarettes

MARIJUANA CIGARETTE/THAI STICK

Visual Description:
A dried, green leafy substance mixed with stems and possibly seeds, hand-rolled into a cigarette (joint).

Methods of Use:
Smoked

Duration of Effects:
Onset: 8-10 Seconds
Peak: 10-30 Minutes
Duration: Variable

Symptoms of Use:
Nystagmus – No
Pupils – Normal (possibly dilated)
Pulse – Elevated
Blood Pressure – Elevated
Body Temperature – Near normal
Non-Convergence – Yes
Bloodshot eyes
Body tremors
Debris in mouth
Difficulty concentrating
Disoriented
Eyelid tremors
Impaired divided attention
Impaired time/distance perception
Increased appetite
Odor of burning marijuana
Rebound dilation
Relaxed inhibitions

Overdose Symptoms:
Fatigue
Paranoia
Psychosis

MARIJUANA GROW

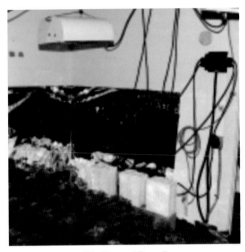

Marijuana "Grow"

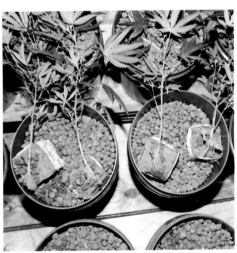

Marijuana "Grow" showing
individual potted plants.

MARIJUANA GROW

To establish evidence for a cultivation charge:

- Photographically document the roots of plants to demonstrate live plant status at time of seizure.
- Document/seize evidence such as weighing devices and articles showing identity of persons in control of premises.
- Outdoor cultivation – pipes (buried or above ground), hoses or other evidence of irrigation systems consistent with marijuana cultivation; other trees, shrubs or plants planted or maintained to hide marijuana plants from view; gardening tools, fertilizer, seeds, sheds/facilities for hanging, drying, processing and packaging for distribution; security devices or systems such as video surveillance, booby traps and armed security personnel.
- Indoor cultivation – grow lights, tubing or hoses or pipes arranged for use as an irrigation system for watering individual plants or maintaining a hydroponic garden; seeds, plant medium, various sizes of pots, foil to cover walls and/or ceilings to reflect light and heat inward (improving growth patterns and/or limiting heat escape); transformers, heating/cooling and lighting systems for cultivation; security systems; facilities for hanging, drying, processing, storing, packaging and mailing of marijuana.
- Also: literature, magazines and computer data regarding cultivation techniques, especially those specific to marijuana; pays and owes regarding distribution of narcotics.
- Computer equipment or electronic storage devices, handwritten notes or printed confidential password lists to enter secured files; indicators of Internet usage and "favorite" or "bookmarked" Internet locations dealing with the use, cultivation and trafficking of marijuana and other narcotics.

Medical Marijuana

The status of "medical marijuana" varies from state to state as to quantities allowed to grow for "Personal Use" and other conditions of use.

HASHISH OIL

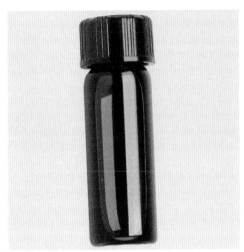

Hash Oil (Dark)

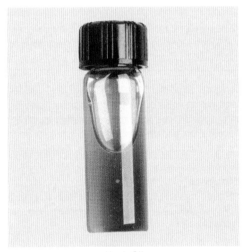

Hash Oil

HASHISH OIL

Visual Description:
Concentrated, thick liquid, dark or gold in color.

Methods of Use:
Smoked - Mixed with tobacco or marijuana.

Effects:
Onset: 8-10 Seconds
Peak: 10-30 Minutes
Duration: 4-6 Hours (variable)

Symptoms:
Nystagmus – No
Pupils – Normal (possibly dilated)
Pulse – Elevated
Blood Pressure – Elevated
Body Temperature – Near normal
Non-Convergence – Yes
Bloodshot eyes
Body tremors
Debris in mouth
Difficulty concentrating
Disoriented
Eyelid tremors
Impaired divided attention
Impaired time/distance perception
Increased appetite
Odor of burning marijuana
Rebound dilation
Relaxed inhibitions

Overdose Symptoms:
Fatigue
Paranoia
Psychosis

HASHISH

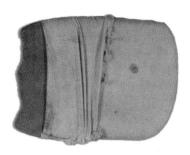

Hashish in bag used for transportation.

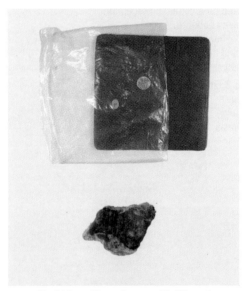

Hashish and bag shown with 10 cent coin for comparison.

HASHISH

Visual Description:
Solid dark green or gold substance.

Methods of Use:
Ingested, Smoked

Effects:
Onset: 8-10 Seconds
Peak: 10-30 Minutes
Duration: 4-6 Hours (variable)

Symptoms:
Nystagmus – No
Pupils – Normal (possibly dilated)
Pulse – Elevated blood pressure
Body Temperature - Near normal
Non-Convergence – Yes
Bloodshot eyes
Body tremors
Debris in mouth
Difficulty concentrating
Disoriented
Eyelid tremors
Impaired divided attention
Impaired time/distance perception
Increased appetite
Odor of burning marijuana
Rebound dilation
Relaxed inhibitions

Overdose Symptoms:
Fatigue
Paranoia
Psychosis

This page intentionally left blank.

DEPRESSANTS

ALCOHOL (ETHANOL)

Visual Description:

Liquid, various odors, colors & flavors. Also found in some perfumes, after-shaves, food flavorings (e.g. vanilla, almond, lemon extracts).

Effects:

Onset: Rapid (varies with quantity consumed and rate of consumption)

Duration: Roughly .02 BAC metabolized per hour.

Method of Use:

Ingested. Some reports of alcohol enemas in college scene. An alcohol inhalation machine (called AWOL for "alcohol without liquid") mixes alcohol with oxygen which is then inhaled. The AWOL concept has gained popularity in Asia and Europe but is meeting resistance in the U.S. and has been banned in some areas.

Symptoms:

Nystagmus – Yes

Pupils – Near normal size, reaction slowed

Pulse – Elevated

Blood Pressure – Elevated

Body Temperature – Subnormal

Non-Convergence – Yes

Euphoria

Lack of coordination

Slurred speech

Exaggerated emotional state

Reduced visual acuity, peripheral vision & glare recovery

Ataxia

Impaired judgment & reflexes

Increased pain threshold

Reduced inhibitions

Boisterous or aggressive behavior

Overdose Symptoms:

Incontinence

Inability to stand or walk

Coma

Respiratory depression

Pulmonary aspiration

Death

ALCOHOL (ETHANOL)

Delirium Tremens (DT's)

May begin within 48-72 hours for chronic heavy abusers who stop their consumption of alcohol.

Additional Comments:

The average adult can metabolize about 7-10 g of alcohol per hour (rate variable per individual and overall blood alcohol level). While tolerance may vary greatly in individuals, generally speaking an ethanol level below 300 mg/dL in a comatose patient presented to the ER will initiate a search for alternative causes (medical condition or other drugs).

Body Fluids Required For Testing:

While breath and blood are the preferred samples for alcohol alone, urine should be considered if other drugs are suspected.

BARBITURATES

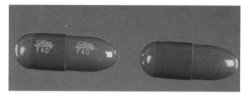

Seconal (secobarbital) Capsules

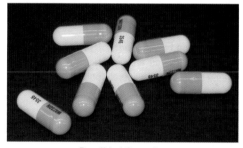

Butalbital Capsules

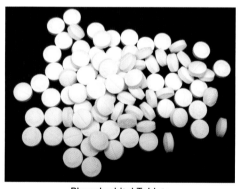

Phenobarbital Tablets

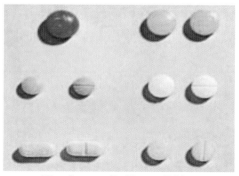

Miscellaneous Barbiturate Tablets

BARBITURATES

Drug Name – Trade Name (representative)
   Amobarbital – Amytal
   Butalbital – Fiorinal or Fioricet
   Mephobarbital – Mebaral
   Pentobarbital – Numbutal
   Phenobarbital – Luminal
   Secobarbital – Seconal, Tuinal
   Butabarbital Sodium – Butisol
   Methohexital – Brevital
   Thiopental – Pentothal

Visual Description:
   Various colored capsules. Most commonly abused are secobarbital (red devils), pentobarbital (yellow jackets) and amobarbital (blue angels).

Methods of Use:
   Ingested, injected, snorted

Duration of Effects:
   1-16 hours depending on which drug taken.

Possible Effects:
   Sedation, hypnosis and/or deep coma
   Anesthesia
   Lethargy
   Slurred speech
   Nystagmus
   Ataxia
   Mild to severe intoxication

Additional Comments:
   Barbiturates range from ultra short acting, such as methohexital and thiopental; to short acting, such as pentobarbital; to intermediate acting, such as amobarbital or butabarbital; to long acting, such as phenobarbital or methobarbital. Typically used as hypnotic/sedative agents, for induction of anesthesia, treatment of epilepsy, and as anticonvulsants.

Special Testing Notes:
   Short/intermediate acting barbiturates may be detected in urine 24-72 hours; longer acting barbiturates up to seven days.

NON-BARBITURATES

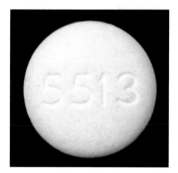

Soma [front]

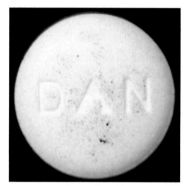

Soma [back]

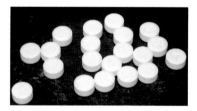

Buspirone 7.5

NON-BARBITURATES

Drug Name – Trade Name (representative)
    Buspirone – BuSpar
    Carisoprodol — Soma
    Chloral hydrate – Noctec, Somnote, Aquachloral, Supprettes
    Ethchlorvynol – Placidyl
    Ethinamate – (no U.S. or Canada brand)
    Glutethimide – Doriden
    Meprobamate – Miltown, Equanil
    Methaqualone – Quaalude
    Methocarbamol – Robaxin
    Methyprylon – Moludar
    Paraldehyde – Paral

Visual Description:
    Various colors and brands of tablets.

Methods of Use:
    Ingested, injected, snorted

Duration of Effects:
    1-16 hours depending on which drug taken.

Possible Effects:
    Sedation, hypnosis and/or deep coma
    Anesthesia
    Lethargy
    Slurred speech
    Nystagmus
    Ataxia
    Mild to severe intoxication

Additional Comments:
    Methaqualone pharmaceutical products were discontinued in 1984 in U.S. May see counterfeit, foreign or old stock.

ANTI-PSYCHOTIC TRANQUILIZERS

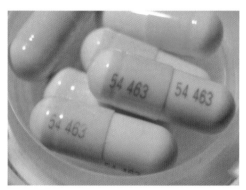

Lithium (Eskalith)

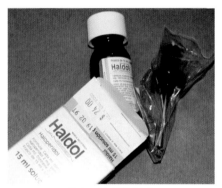

Halperidol (Haldol)

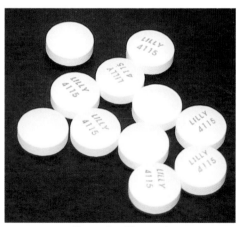

Olenzapine (Zyprexa)

ANTI-PSYCHOTIC TRANQUILIZERS

Drug Name – Trade Name (representative)
- **Chlorpromazine** – Thorazine
- **Clozapine** – Clozaril
- **Droperidol** – Inapsine
- **Fluphenazine HCl** – Prolixin
- **Haloperidol** – Haldol
- **Lithium** – Eskalith, Lithobid, Lithane (Canada)
- **Loxapine** – Loxitane
- **Mesoridazine** – Serentil
- **Molindone** – Moban
- **Olanzapine** – Zyprexa
- **Perphenazine** – Trilafon
- **Prochlorperazine** – Compazine
- **Promethazine** – Phenergan
- **Risperidone** – Risperdal
- **Seroquel** – Quetiapine Fumarate
- **Thioridazine** – Mellaril
- **Trimethobenzamide** – Tigan

Visual Description:
Various Tablets

Methods of Use:
Ingested, Snorted

Possible Symptoms:
Mild to severe intoxication, sedation, dry mouth (Exception: Clozapine can cause hypersalivation)
Absence of sweating
Tachycardia
Coma
Seizures
Jaw muscle spasm
Rigidity
Respiratory arrest
Either hypothermia or hyperthermia may be seen.
Overdose may be seen in suicide attempts though some are not extremely toxic.

BENZODIAZEPINES
(Benzo)

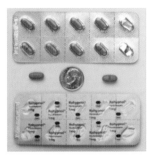

Flunitrazepam (Rohypnol)

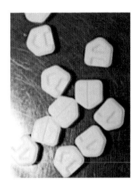

Lorazepam (Ativan)

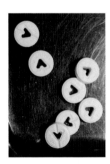

Diazepam (Valium)

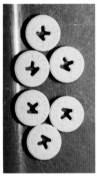

Clonazepam
(Klonopin or Rivotril [Mexico])

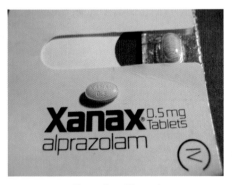

Alprazolam (Xanax)

BENZODIAZEPINES
(Benzo)

Drug Name – Trade Name (representative)

Alprazolam – Xanax, Niravam
Bromazepam – Lexotan (Mexico)
Chlordiazepoxide – Librium
Clonazepam – Klonopin or Rivotril (Mexico)
Clorazepate – Tranzene
Diazepam – Valium
Estazolam – ProSom
Flunitrazepam – Rohypnol (aka: roofies)
Flurazepam – Dalmane
Halazepam – Paxipam
Lorazepam – Ativan
Midazolam – Versed
Nimetazepam – Erimin (Asian)
Nitrazepam – Mogadan
Oxazepam – Serax
Phenazepam - (Russian)
Prazepam – Centrax
Quazepam – Doral
Temazepam – Restoril
Triazolam – Halcion

Visual Description:
Various tablets; may be ground up for snorting. Used to dose others for rape or robbery; may be powder or dissolved into liquid (in small vial or nasal spray or eye drop container).

Methods of Use:
Ingested, Injected, Snorted

Possible Effects:
Benzodiazepine drugs give a wide range of typical CNS depressant effects. Typically used as anti-anxiety tranquilizers, sleep aids, withdrawal treatment for other drugs, seizure medications, etc. Causes sedation, blurred vision, drowsiness, lethargy, ataxia, fatigue, mental depression, loss of coordination, hypotension, diminished reflexes, confusion, coma, etc. Hypothermia possible.

Special Testing Note:
Some of these drugs are difficult to capture in testing. Some may not show up in a drug "screen" and require further testing. Triazolam and prazepam are particularly difficult to detect. Newer benzodiazepines or low concentrations may not be detected.

Additional Comments:
Flunitrazepam (Rohypnol) and bromazepam (Lexotan) are not approved for use in the United States but are commonly smuggled into the U.S. for abuse purposes, especially from Mexico. Foreign prescriptions for flunitrazepam are not honored in the U.S.

GHB/XYREM/GBL/BD/OTHER ANALOGS
(Depressant/Dissociative Anesthetic)

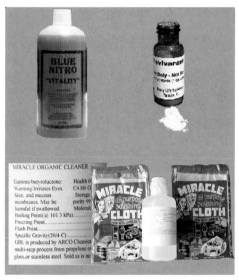

Miscellaneous forms of GBL.

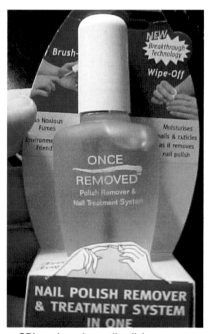

GBL packaged as nail polish remover.

GHB/XYREM/GBL/BD/OTHER ANALOGS
(Depressant/Dissociative Anesthetic)

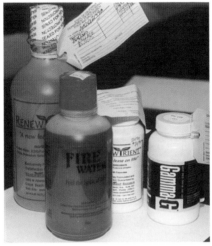

GHB Analogs

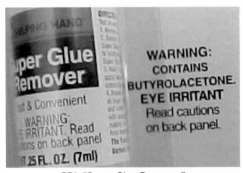

GBL "Super Glue Remover"

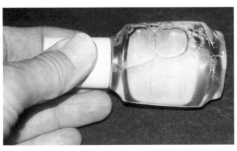

GHB "Mouthwash"

GHB/XYREM/GBL/BD/OTHER ANALOGS
(Depressant/Dissociative Anesthetic)

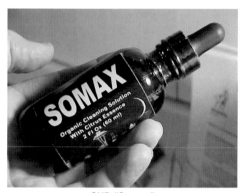

GHB "Somax"

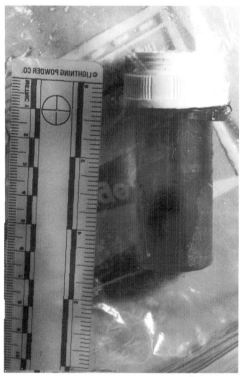

GHB packaged as evidence.

GHB/XYREM/GBL/BD/OTHER ANALOGS
(Depressant/Dissociative Anesthetic)

Visual Description:
Commonly liquid, various textures; clear or yellowish color. Often colored for disguise or to avoid accidental consumption. No distinguishing odor – from mild chemical odor to nasty smell. Salty taste, but masked by sweet/fruity drinks. May see powder or capsules. Hydroscopic – likely to become moist if exposed to damp air.

Methods of Use:
Ingested. Reported rectal insertion of GHB-soaked tampons, called "teabagging."

Duration of Effects:
Onset: 10-20 minutes (some analogs slightly slower)
Duration: 3-5 hours

Possible Symptoms:
Nystagmus – Vertical usually present (may be absent in low levels)
Pupils – Slow to react; near normal size
Pulse/Blood Pressure – generally lowered, may be high (not consistent)
Body Temperature – Near normal to low
Non-Convergence - Yes
Dizziness
Lack of facial expression (blank stare)
Droopy eyelids (Ptosis)
Amnesia
Vomiting/nausea
Aggression/combativeness or sexual stimulation possible
Drunken behavior (without odor of alcohol)
Muscle tone from flaccid to periods of rigidity
Sudden resolution of symptoms (after approx 4 hours)

Overdose Symptoms:
Loss of bowel and urinary control   Pulmonary edema
Cold & clammy skin   Death
Coma
Shallow respiration (may drop to only 5-6 times per minute)

Special Testing Issues:
GHB is in blood 3-5 hours and urine approximately 12 hours

Associated Chemical/Analog Names
Gamma hydroxybutyrate (GHB); gamma butyrolactone (GBL); 1,4 butanediol (BD or BDO); pyrrolidone; gamma valerolactone (GVL); gamma hydroxyvalerate (GHV); octanediol; tetrahydrofuranone; tetramethylene glycol.

MISCELLANEOUS DEPRESSANTS

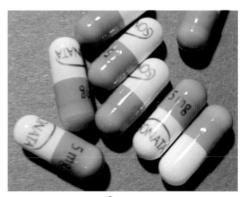

Sonata

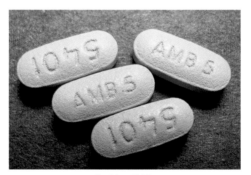

Ambien 5 Mg

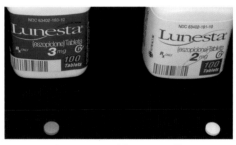

Lunesta 3mg (r) and 2mg (l)

MISCELLANEOUS DEPRESSANTS

ANTIHISTAMINES
Diphenhydramine HCl - Benadryl
Hydroxyzine - Vistaral, Atarax, Pliva (Vet use)

SLEEPING MEDICATIONS
Eszopiclone - Lunesta
Zaleplon - Sonata
Zolpidem - Ambien

Additional Comments:
While diphenhydramine is a common over-the-counter ingredient, it is impairing for purposes of driving and for use in drugging for robbery or rape, etc. Ambien has been identified in a number of drug rape cases and has been associated with "sleep driving" incidents of DUI and other sleep-walking incidents in which the person has no recall of the conduct. Any drug that causes amnesia or unconsciousness or confusion could be utilized for robbery or rape.

ANTI-DEPRESSANTS

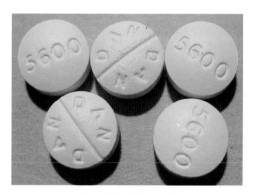

Trazadone (Desyrel)

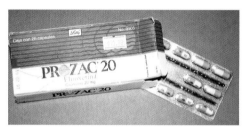

Fluoxetine (Prozac)

ANTI-DEPRESSANTS

Drug Name – Trade Name (representative)
Amitriptyline HCI – Elavil
Amoxapine – Asendin
Bupropion – Wellbutrin, Zyban
Citalopram HCI – Celexa
Clomipramine – Anafranil
Desipramine – Norpramine
Doxepin HCI – Sinequan
Escitalopram – Lexapro
Fluoxetine – Prozac
Fluvoxamine – Luvox
Imipramine – Rofranil
Isocarboxazide – Marplan
Maprotiline – Ludiomil
Mirtazapine – Remeron
Nefazodone – Serzone
Nortriptyline – Aventyl or Pamelor
Paroxetine – Paxil
Phenelzine – Nardil
Protryptaline – Vivactil, Triptil (Canada)
Sertraline HCI – Zoloft
Tranylcypromine – Pamate
Trazadone – Desyrel
Trimipramine – Surmontil, Apo-Trimip (Canada)
Venlafaxine – Effexor

Visual Description:
Various

Methods of Use:
Ingested, Injected, Snorted

Possible Effects:
Overdose may cause ataxia, sedation, seizures, coma. Can produce restlessness, anxiety and agitation, especially Bupropion. Mirtazapine (Remeron) has a prominent sedative effect.

Additional Comments:
Noncyclic anti-depressants such as Desyrel, Serzone, Prozac, Zoloft, Paxil, Luvox, Effexor and Wellbutrin, are typically less toxic than the tricyclics, such as Elavil, Asendin, Anafranil, Sinequan, Rofranil, Ludiomil, Aventyl, etc. Tricyclics are sometimes used in suicidal overdoses and represent a significant cause of poisoning in hospitalizations and deaths.

These drugs are listed in the DEPRESSANTS category based on their overall action of depressing the body's central nervous system. The term "anti-depressants" refers to the action of the drugs in adjusting the user's mental mood. The FDA now requires most anti-depressant medications to warn that these drugs may increase risks of suicidal thinking and behavior, especially in young adults during the first few months of treatment.

This page intentionally left blank.

HALLUCINOGENS

PHENETHYLAMINES

2C-B — 4-bromo-2,5-dimethoxyphenethylamine
(Bromo, Nexus)

2C-E — 2,5 dimethoxy-4-ethylphenethylamine

2C-I — 2,5-dimethoxy-4-iodophenethylamine

2C-T-7 — 2,5-dimethoxy-4-(n)-propylthiophenethylamine
(Lucky 7, Tripstacy)

2-TOM — 5-methoxy-4-methyl-2-methylthioamphetamine

3C-BZ — 4-benzyloxy-3,5-dimethoxyamphetamine

3C-E — 3,5-dimethoxy-4-ethoxyamphetamine

5-TOM — 2-methoxy-4-methyl-5-methylthio-A

DOB — 4-bromo-2,5-dimethoxyamphetamine

DOC — 4-chloro-2,5-dimethoxyamphetamine (analog of DOB)

MDA — 3,4 methylenedioxy-amphetamine

MDMA — 3,4 methylenedioxy-methamphetamine
(See MDMA, Ecstasy, page 38)

Additional Comments:
There are at least 179 drugs in the category. 2C-B and 2C-I are the most common, after MDMA and MDA. But there are others such as:
2C-C, 2C-D, 2C-E, 2C-G, 2C-G-5, 2C-N, 2C-P, 2C-T, 2C-T-2, 2C-T-4, 2C-T-5, 2C-T-8, 2C-T-9, 3C-BZ, 2-4-DMA, DOM, HOT-2, 4-MA, MDDM, MDBZ, MDMC, MEDA, MMDA, 4-TIM, TMA-4, 4-T-TRIS

Visual Description:
Powder or pills, various colors and shapes; with or without logo imprints; DOC & DOB also seen as liquid in vials and blotter paper, resembling LSD format

Methods of Use:
Ingested primarily as pills. May be snorted, injected or inserted rectally

Duration of Effects:
Varies greatly with the substance taken

Possible Effects:

Pupils – Dilated	**Pulse** – Elevated
Blood Pressure – Elevated	**Body Temperature** – Elevated

These drugs are generally hallucinogenic stimulants but with varying effects. Some are more hallucinogenic and some are more stimulant oriented. The effects will be somewhat similar to both categories.

Familiarity with this class of drugs is rather limited. Law enforcement, and even medical professionals, often have to refer to www.erowid.org for information about usage and effects. Much of the material on that pro-drug website is obtained from Dr. Alex Shulgin, known as Papa Ecstasy, who created many of these drugs and has taken and documented all of them as well. A wider variety of these drugs is showing up with increasing frequency. Many are currently scheduled but many are not. Some may be covered as analogs of scheduled drugs. Contact your crime lab or DEA for the legal status in your state.

MDMA - PHENETHYLAMINES

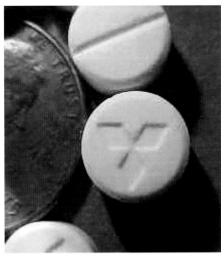

"Mitsubishi" MDMA
(shown with penny for size comparison)

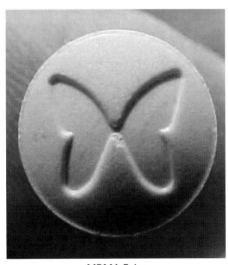

MDMA Fake

Actually Remifeminin, a harmless dietary supplement that happens to have a butterfly imprint and has been seen sold as Ecstasy. This product has the butterfly on both sides, rare for an actual MDMA pill.

(cont'd next pg.)

MDMA - PHENETHYLAMINES

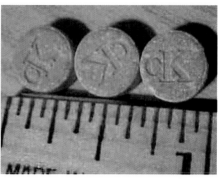

MDMA with Calvin Klein "brand"

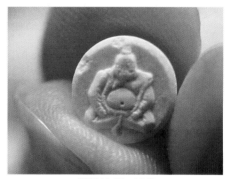

MDMA "Budda"

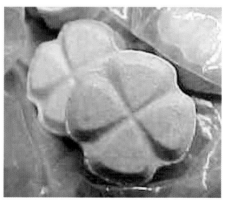

MDMA "Green Clover"

MDMA - PHENETHYLAMINES

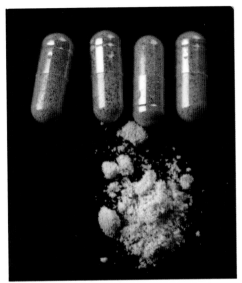

MDMA Capsules

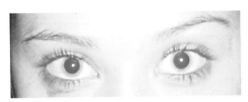

MDMA User
(Note extremely dilated pupils)

(cont'd next pg.)

MDMA - PHENETHYLAMINES
MDMA — 3,4 METHYLENEDIOXYMETHAMPHETAMINE
(Ecstasy, X, XTC, E, The Hug Drug)
MDA – 3,4 METHYLENEDIOXY-AMPHETAMINE
(Phenethylamine)

Visual Description:
White or off-white powder or pills. Pills may appear professionally pressed or coarse, homemade. May be a variety of shapes and colors. Seen plain (no logo) or any of 600 cartoons characters, business logos (Mitsubishi, Nike, etc), or symbols (heart, happy face, etc.) Price of a pill varies from $15 to $40; wholesale $6 to $9. (See Paraphernalia, pg. 144)

Methods of Use:
Ingested primarily as pills. May be snorted, injected or inserted rectally.

Duration of Effects:
Onset: 25-40 minutes
Duration: 4-6 hours desired effects
Impaired for driving up to 12 hours: may have intense fatigue afterwards.

Possible Effects:
Nystagmus – Yes
Pupils – Dilated (large)
Pulse – Elevated
Blood Pressure – Elevated
Body Temperature – Elevated
Non-Convergence – No
Altered perception (visual alterations; true hallucinations not likely); altered sense of time.
Anxiety
Blurred vision
Bruxism
Chills or sweating
Decreased aggression (unless used poly drug or in high doses)
Depression (after effects wear off or with long-term use)
Dry mouth
Enhanced sense of smell, touch, taste, sight
Enhanced energy; hyperactive
Euphoria
Faintness
Greater self esteem (temporary)
Increased communication (talkative and open)
Lack of inhibitions
Nausea
Paranoia
Sensation of loving all and being loved by all
Sweating

MDMA - PHENETHYLAMINES

Overdose Symptoms:
   Body temperature out of control
   Bizarre behavior
   Coma
   Psychosis
   Death

Additional Comments:

"Ecstasy" has become virtually an umbrella term for a variety of substances in that pills sold as such may contain little or no MDMA (Ecstasy). Related substances (see pages on tryptamines and phenethylamines) may be substituted or included in the pill content. Or the pill may contain meth (for stimulant effect) and LSD or PCP or mescaline (to provide hallucinogenic effect) to simulate MDMA. Or the pill may contain over-the-counter substances such as dextromethorphan (DXM, cough suppressant), ephedrine, or simply pure bunk. The content of MDMA in actual MDMA pills may vary from 50 to 175 mgs (typical pill size is around 300 mgs). Key ingredient for MDMA is safrole (iso-safrole, bromo-safrole or chloro-safrole).

MDA provides more visual disturbance than MDMA and isn't quite as popular. Many of the pills sold as Ecstasy contain only MDA or MDA mixed with other drugs. It should be noted that MDA is also a breakdown product of MDMA in the body. Toxicology results may show a ratio of MDMA to MDA as roughly 85 to 15. That does not in itself indicate ingestion of MDA, but rather ingestion of MDMA metabolizing.

There are more than 600 recognized logos on Ecstasy pills, cartoon characters, business logos, letters, etc. Thus there are many nicknames, typically based on the logo and color or shape of the pill. They do not symbolize a particular dealer or maker. One pill press can produce a variety of logos daily as the metal die with the logo imprint can be readily changed through a pill run.

Death from heatstroke type of event can occur. Users dehydrate and are trained to drink large amounts of water, but excessive water intake during this period can also result in death from hyponatremia, water poisoning.

TRYPTAMINES

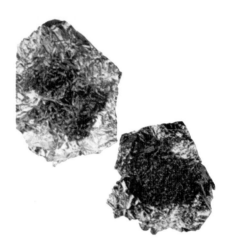

DMT in Foil Bindles

TRYPTAMINES

AMT – Alpha-methyl-tryptamine or Spirals, Amtrak or Amthrax
5-MeO-DIPT — 5-methoxy-N,N-diisopropyltryptamine or
  Foxy or Foxy Methoxy
DMT – Dimethyltryptamine (DMT photo on previous page)

There are at least 55 drugs in this category. Most tryptamines occur in nature but all are also synthetically produced. Tryptamines include: **2-Me-DET, 2-Me-DMT, 4-MeO-DIPT, 4-HO-MIPT, 4-HO-DBT, 5-MeO-DMT, DIPT, MBT, 4,5-MDO-DIPT, MBT, AET, DET (analog of DMT)**

Tryptamines commonly recognized as drugs of abuse (but perhaps not commonly known as tryptamines) include Psilocybin (O-phosphoryl-4-hydroxy-N,N-dimethyltryptamine) and psilocyn (4-hydroxy-N, N-dimethyltryptamine) and even LSD.

Visual Description:
  Powder or pills, various colors and shapes; with or without logo imprints. AMT is often seen in pills with the oval alien face or spider imprint. Foxy has been found in off-white or orange crystal powder or in capsule or tablet form.

Methods of Use:
  Ingested primarily as pills. May be snorted, injected, inserted rectally or smoked.

Duration of Effects:
  Varies greatly with the substance taken. AMT lasts 12-24 hours. Foxy 3-6 hours.

Possible Effects:
  Pupils – Dilated
  Pulse – Elevated
  Blood Pressure – Elevated
  Body Temperature – Elevated
  Visual and auditory distortions
  Emotional disturbances

These drugs are hallucinogenic stimulants but with varying effects. Some are more hallucinogenic and some are more stimulant oriented. The effects will be somewhat similar to both categories.

Additional Comments:
Familiarity with this class of drugs is rather limited. Law enforcement and even medical professionals often have to refer to *erowid.org* for information about usage and effects. Much of the material on that pro-drug website is obtained from Dr. Alex Shulgin, known as Papa Ecstasy, who created many of these drugs and has taken and documented all of them as well.

(cont'd next pg.)

TRYPTAMINES

DMT (DIMETHYLTRYPTAMINE), also known as the "Businessman's Lunch" is one of the most commonly abused tryptamines. It is commonly found in crystalline form, powder or oil, and varies from white to pink to red, w/smell when heated similar to burning plastic

DMT May be snorted, smoked as vapor or mixed with tobacco, marijuana, etc. and smoked, injected, and the effects last approximately 45-60 minutes

Possible Effects:

> **Pupils** – Dilated
> **Pulse** – Elevated
> **Blood Pressure** – Elevated
> **Body Temperature** – Elevated
> Blank stareMood changes

Body tremors	Muscle tension
Dazed	Nausea
Disoriented	Perspiring
Flashbacks	Sleeplessness
Hallucinations	Synesthesia
Memory loss	

Overdose Symptoms:

> Bizarre behavior
> Long, intense trips
> Psychosis
> Death

Additional Comments:

5-MeO-DMT (5-methoxy-N,N-dimethyl- tryptamine) is related to DMT and comes from certain plants or is synthesized. Smoked or snorted. It is one of the two ingredients excreted by the Bufo Alvarius toad (indigenous to southwestern areas of U.S.). This toad excretes venom from glands on its back, containing hallucinogenic substances bufotenine and 5-MeO-DMT. Collected by squeezing the glands; smoke the dried extract. Popularized by the media as licking the toad's back (scaring it first to cause excretion). A wider variety of these drugs is showing up with increasing frequency. Many are currently scheduled, but many are not. Some may be covered as analogs of scheduled drugs. Contact your crime lab or DEA for the legal status in your state.

This page intentionally left blank.

JIMSON WEED
Datura

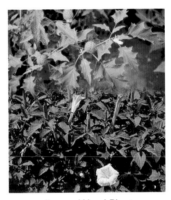

Jimson Weed Plant

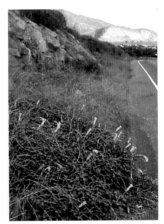

Jimson Weed Growing Wild

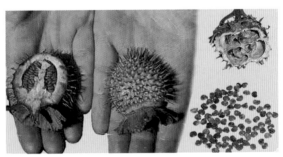

Jimson Weed Pod and Seeds

JIMSON WEED
Datura

Visual Description:
Green bush with white trumpet shaped flowers (can range white to purple). The flower pods contain seeds that are consumed. When dried, the pods are light green in color and prickly.

Methods of Use:
Eaten or ingested as tea or smoked

Duration of Effects:
Variable

Possible Effects:
Nystagmus – No
Pupils – Dilated
Pulse – Elevated
Blood Pressure – Elevated
Body Temperature – Elevated
Non-Convergence – No
Blank stare
Body tremors
Delirium
Disoriented
Hallucinations
Impaired divided attention
Mood changes
Memory loss
Muscle tension
Nausea
Perspiring
Sleeplessness
Synesthesia

Overdose Symptoms:
Bizarre behavior
Psychosis
Violence
Death

Additional Comments:
Also called angel's trumpet, devil's trumpet, moon flower and Jamestown weed. Active ingredients are the alkaloids hyoscyamine, scopolamine and atropine. Can be very toxic and resulting behavior can be very dangerous.

LSD
Lysergic Acid Diethylamide

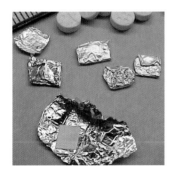 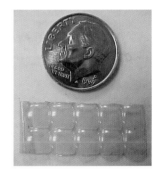

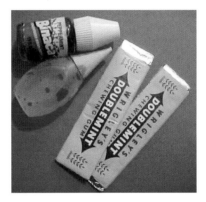

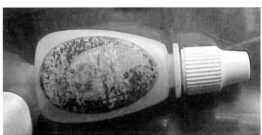

Various Forms of LSD

LSD
Lysergic Acid Diethylamide

Visual Description:
Varies – Pure crystals typically clear or white; traditional blotter paper (small squares, perforated sheets, or strips of impregnated paper, often with cartoon characters or artistic designs); on a sugar cube; often seen as a liquid (in small vials such as breath mint, eye or nasal spray, food coloring containers); in gel form as dots on plastic pieces that are sucked; gel form as "pyramids" on, or peeled from, fluorescent light diffuser plastic (used as a mold and then peeled off and cut into strips or perforated first, broken into pieces and sucked). May also be mixed in tablets sold as "Ecstasy" (may contain meth and LSD, if actual MDMA isn't available to achieve similar effects of hallucinogenic stimulant).

Methods of Use:
Ingested; absorbed (skin contact or eye drops). Tiny quantities when in crystalline form (50 micrograms = one hit). Cannot be smoked (destroyed by heat). One ounce of pure LSD equals 567,000 hits, calculated at 50 micrograms each.

Duration of Effects:
Onset: 20-60 minutes
Duration: 6-12 hours

Possible Symptoms:
Nystagmus – No
Pupils – Dilated
Pulse – Elevated
Blood Pressure – Elevated
Body Temperature – Elevated
Non-Convergence – No

Ataxia	Impaired sense of time & distance
Anxiety (bad trip)	Increased salivation
Blank stare	Muscle tension
Dazed, disoriented, delirium	Nausea
Fear & paranoia (bad trip)	Perspiring
Flashbacks	Piloerection (goosebumps)
Hyperthermia (overheating)	Psychosis
Impaired divided attention	Synesthesia
Sleeplessness	

Additional Comments:
Synesthesia is a condition where one type of stimulation evokes the sensation of another, as when the hearing of a sound produces the visualization of a color)

LSA
D-Lysergic Acid Amide

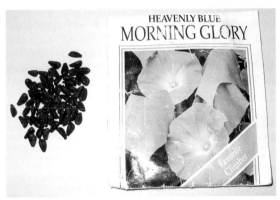

Morning Glory Seeds, Hawaiian Woodrose Seeds

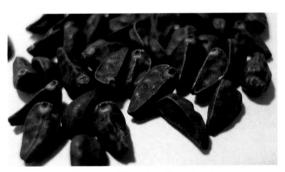

Close-up of Morning Glory Seeds

LSA
D-Lysergic Acid Amide

Visual Description:

Seeds from Morning Glory (produces variety of flower colors), Hawaiian Woodrose, and Stipa robusta plants, plus ergot fungus.

Methods of Use:

Suck on or swallow seeds.

Grind and soak the seeds and drink the liquid.

Brew tea.

Duration of Effects & Possible Effects:

See LSD; LSA provides similar effects though typically milder.

Additional Comments:

This chemical is used in synthesizing LSD. Gives a milder version of an LSD trip.

PEYOTE
Peyote Cactus – Mescaline

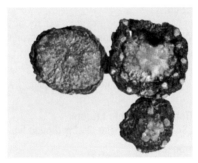

Peyote Button

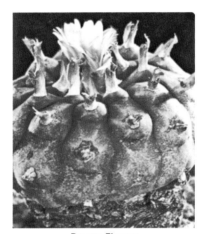

Peyote Flower

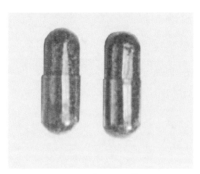

Peyote in Capsule Form

PEYOTE
Peyote Cactus – Mescaline

Visual Description:
Capsules (gelatin capsules of ground plant material or white crystalline powder if synthesized), needle-shaped translucent crystals, hard brown discs of plant material (the "button" from the plant is removed and dried), tablets.

Methods of Use:
Ingested as capsules or tablets or in soup or tea form; chewed; smoked.

Duration of Effects:
Onset: 30-60 minutes
Duration: 10-12 hours

Possible Symptoms:
Nystagmus – No
Pupils – Dilated
Pulse – Elevated
Blood Pressure – Elevated
Body Temperature – Elevated
Non-Convergence – No
Ataxia
Dazed/disoriented
Hallucinations
Memory loss
Psychosis
Rancid breath
Synesthesia
Sweating
Nausea/vomiting

Additional Comments:
Not illegal for certain members of the Native American Church; used for religious purposes. Documentation of tribal membership and authorization may be required for possession and transportation; verify requirements and department policy in your region.

PSILOCYBIN & PSILOCIN
(Magic Mushrooms)

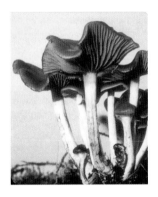 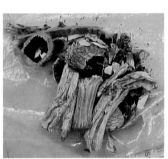

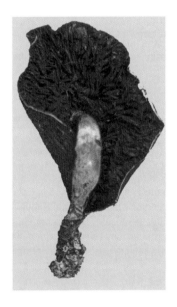

PSILOCYBIN & PSILOCIN
(Magic Mushrooms)

Visual Description:
Fresh or dried mushrooms (only specific plants); white to brown powder or capsules. Usually stored dry to avoid mold and spoiling.

Methods of Use:
Chewed as plant material, swallowed as a capsule or consumed as tea, ground and smoked mixed with marijuana

Duration of Effects:
Onset: within 20 minutes
Duration: 6-12 Hours

Possible Effects:
Nystagmus – No
Pupils – Dilated
Pulse – Elevated
Blood Pressure – Elevated
Body Temperature – Elevated
Non-Convergence – No

Abdominal pain	Impaired concentration & perception
Ataxia	Muscle tension & twitching
Chills	Nausea
Dazed/Disoriented	Numbness of face, tongue or lips
Difficult/Tremulous speech	Synesthesia
Dizziness	Sleeplessness
Euphoria	Slowed passage of time
Fever & Flushing	Psychosis
Hallucinations	Urinary incontinence
Hypertension	Vomiting
Visualization of patterns with eyes closed	

Additional Comments:
Growing magic mushrooms for profit is typically a very high-tech operation with growing beds, elaborate conditions, sterilized fertilizer material, etc. Some mushrooms that may be mistaken for "magic mushrooms" are poisonous. Amanita muscaria mushrooms contain the substances ibotenic acid and muscimol (rather than psilocybin and psilocin), causing similar hallucinogenic reactions but may also be fatal. They have a brown, red or orange cap with white "warts."

SALVIA DIVINORUM

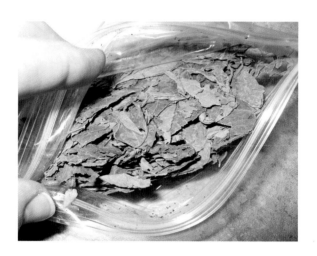

SALVIA DIVINORUM

Visual Description:

Green plant material (seeds are uncommon; produced from plant cuttings most often). A sage type plant from the mint family. The active ingredient is Salvinorin A)

Methods of Use:

Chewing leaves or drinking tea or soup concoction or smoking. May mix with honey and eat by spoonfuls.

Duration of Effects:

Onset: One minute
Peak: 5-10 minutes
Duration: One hour (Impairment for driving likely for several hours)

Possible Symptoms:

Abdominal pain
Diarrhea
Difficulty communicating or unable
Euphoria
Hallucinations
Headache/Hangover
Intoxication
Meditative or trance state
Sweaty
Terrifying experiences possible
Uncontrolled laughter at onset
Vomiting
Visual disturbances

Additional Comments:

Salvia Divinorum, as of 2008, has been banned at various levels by at least 12 states (Delaware, Florida, Illinois, Kansas, Mississippi, Missouri, North Dakota, Oklahoma, Virginia, Tennessee, Louisiana, Maine) with legislation pending in several others, and is being considered for federal legislation. Research is being reviewed. Some other countries have banned it as well. More hallucinogenic than marijuana and somewhat similar to ingestion of Datura (Jimson Weed), legislation is needed in every state. Sold under such names as "purple sticky," 10X, 20X, 30X, Happy-Smoke and Maria Pastora in head shops around the country and on the Internet.

NUTMEG – MYRISTICIN
3-Methoxy-4,5-methylene-dioxyallybenzene and Related Compounds

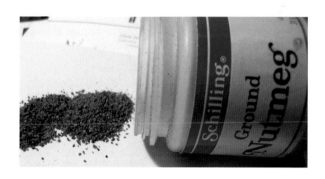

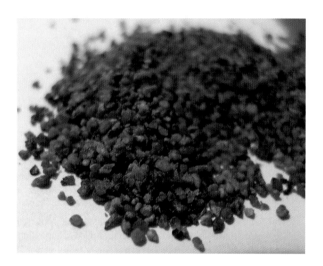

NUTMEG – MYRISTICIN
3-Methoxy-4,5-methylene-dioxyallybenzene
and Related Compounds

Visual Description:
Dried kernel of the myristica fragrans tree, ground for use as a spice.

Methods of Use:
Ingested; usually mixed with liquid to avoid chewing. Some recommend trying to swallow it dry while others recommend orange juice and honey and other recommend frozen concoctions with ice and lemonade. Requires fairly large amounts, such as multiple tablespoons. One pro-drug website nutmeg user recommends 15 grams for a 150 pound person as a starting point, for example.

Duration of Effects:
Onset: From 2 to 8 hours after ingestion
Duration: 24 hours, with minor effects up to 48-72 hours

Possible Effects:
Nystagmus – No
Pupils – Dilated
Pulse – Elevated
Blood Pressure – Elevated
Body Temperature – Elevated
Non-Convergence – No

Ataxia	Hypothermia
Constipation	Nausea
Delirium	Psychosis
Diarrhea	Synesthesia
Dry mouth	Sleepiness afterwards
Euphoria	Tachycardia
Flushing	Vomiting
Hallucinations	

Additional Comments:
Though not illegal, nutmeg is often banned from correctional institution kitchens. Not widely abused due to more negative than positive effects, but accessible to youth who seek drug experience. Impairs the ability to drive a motor vehicle.

MISCELLANEOUS HALLUCINOGENIC STIMULANTS

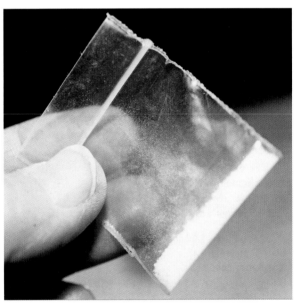

Many of these more unusual drugs (TFMPP, BZP, Euphoria and some of the phenethylamines and tryptamines) are seen as powder or crystal form or may be found pressed into pills just like MDMA (Ecstasy) in appearance. The powders may be in nondescript baggies or in vials or bags labeled as "research chemicals."

MISCELLANEOUS HALLUCINOGENIC STIMULANTS
4-METHYLAMINOREX
(Aka: Euphoria, U4EUH or "Ice")

Chemical name:
4,5-dihydro-4-methyl-5-phenyl-2-oxazolamine

Duration of Effects:
Onset: 1-2 hours
Duration: 14-16 hours

Effects:
Intense stimulant with sensations of boundless energy and mental acuity. Enhanced sense of self-esteem. Described by some as a long-lasting MDMA intoxication superimposed with methamphetamine. Other effects: increased respiration, tachycardia, tremors, perspiration, increased blood pressure, intraocular pressure, blurred vision, tightness in the chest, increased body and breath odor. Has not become particularly popular, likely due to the excessiveness of its effects.

PIPERAZINES — BZP, TFMPP
BENZYLPIPERAZINE (BZP)

Sold as a substitute for Ecstasy, MDMA, BZP is a stimulant with some expanded properties, somewhat similar to MDMA, but also with more undesirable side effects. BZP is federally scheduled. Known as "Poor Man's Ecstasy." Effects last 6-8 hours.

Another piperazine surfaced in 2007. The chemical, 1-(chlorophenyl) piperazine (aka: meta-chlorophenylpiperazine or mCPP) was the major component of pills resembling the usual MDMA pill format. The pills contained only traces of MDMA. BZP is federally scheduled.

TRIFLUOROMETHYLPHENYLPIPERAZINE (TFMPP)

Seen sometimes on its own or mixed with BZP and sold as a recreational drug that is a "legal alternative" to MDMA and/or LSD. Little is known about TFMPP effects. Like BZP it is a stimulant with additional properties. TFMPP is *not* federally scheduled and is sometimes sold as a legal alternative to LSD and MDMA.

While BZP & TFMPP have been the common piperazines of abuse, others have been found in recent times. The piperazine 1-(3-chlorophenyl) piperazine, also known as meta-chlorophenyl piperazine or mCPP), appeared in pill format in a 2007 law enforcement seizure in Indiana. The piperazine 1(2-methoxyphenyl)-piperazine, or OMPP, appeared in a Texas seizure.

This page intentionally left blank.

INHALANTS

INHALANT ABUSE (GENERAL)

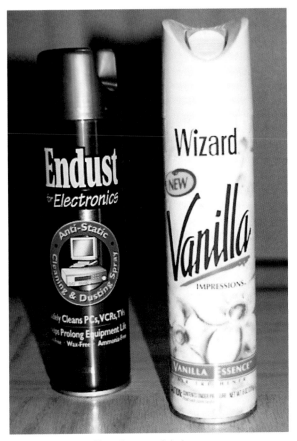

Two Common Inhalants

INHALANT ABUSE (GENERAL)

Four categories of inhalants:

Solvents — Toluene products, paint/paint thinner, lighter fluid, carburetor cleaner, dry cleaning fluid, correction fluid (some brands), household glue/cement, felt-tip markers, gasoline (benzene), kerosene, fingernail polish remover, grease/spot remover (methylene chloride and toluene)

Aerosols — Spray paint, deodorant, body sprays, room odorizer, hair spray, fabric protector, vegetable cooking spray

Gases — Butane, nitrous oxide and other medical anesthetics (ether, chloroform, halothane), propane, helium, freon

Nitrites — amyl (some medical use re angina), butyl nitrite (video head cleaner), cyclohexyl nitritem (Note: Nitrites are slightly different as they primarily dilate blood vessels and relax the muscles and thus are primarily used as sexual enhancers)

Visual Description:

There are more than 1400 volatile, potentially abusable products on the market today, including hydrocarbons, nitrites, anesthetics, alcohols, and halogen compounds. They are called volatile organic compounds (**VOC**). They are products never meant for human consumption, such as butane, fabric protector, gasoline, spray paint, hair spray, marking pens, air fresheners, computer keyboard sprays, cleaning agents, starter fluid, fire extinguisher (halon) and glue. Some are inhaled for the named product itself (such as gasoline, glue) while others are abused for the propellant that releases the product (such as nitrous oxide that fires homemade whipped cream makers and propels whipped cream from store-bought cans and cardiac synthesizers that propel air freshener from their containers).

Methods of Use:

Inhaled from a cloth or bag or balloon, or directly from the container

Duration of Effects:

Onset: Rapid
Duration: Brief

(cont'd next pg.)

INHALANT ABUSE (GENERAL)

Possible Symptoms (varies with substance) and Signs:
>**Nystagmus** – Varies
>**Pupils** – Normal or dilated
>**Pulse** – May be elevated
>**Blood Pressure** – May be elevated
>**Body Temperature** – Varies with substance
>**Non-Convergence** – Possibly
>Acute confusion
>Agitation
>Ataxia
>Brain Damage (especially with long-term use)
>Brief euphoria
>Cardiac arrhythmia/failure (especially with fluorocarbons)
>Decrease in appetite
>Headaches
>Liver & kidney damage possible
>Odor of substance
>Poor memory
>Shortness of breath/chest pains
>Slurred speech
>Stains on clothing or skin
>Sores/rash around mouth/nose
>Suicide risk (with persistent use)
>Sullen/lethargic moods
>Tremors
>Vomiting

Overdose Symptoms:
>Coma
>Death

Additional Comments:
>Long-term use can cause weight loss, fatigue, muscle fatigue. Consistent inhaling of vapors can, over time, permanently damage the nervous system. Inhaling while driving is particularly dangerous and has resulted in traffic accidents and deaths. Another indicator is hidden, excessive numbers of spray product containers, chemical-soaked rags or clothing. Testing is difficult due to the brief time period for most of these products.

This page intentionally left blank.

AMYL/BUTYL NITRITE
CYCLOHEXYL NITRITE

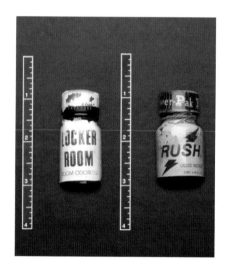

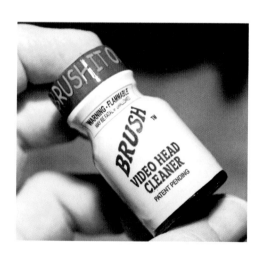

AMYL/BUTYL NITRITE
CYCLOHEXYL NITRITE

Visual Description:
Packaged in small bottles, sold as room deodorizers, video head cleaner, etc. Often called "Locker Room," "Rush," "Come," "Brush," etc.

Methods of Use:
Vapors Inhaled

Duration of Effects:
Onset: Rapid
Duration: 2-5 minutes

Possible Symptoms:
Pupils – May be normal or dilated
Pulse – Elevated
Blood Pressure – May be lowered (due to effect of dilating blood vessels)
Body Temperature – May be elevated
Non-Convergence – Possible
Confusion
Disoriented
Flushed head and neck
Headaches
Odor of substance
Slurred speech
Sudden "head rush"

Overdose Symptoms:
Asphyxiation (buildup of inhaled fumes, displacing oxygen in lungs)
Coma
Death

Additional Comments:
Long-term use can cause weight loss, fatigue, muscle fatigue. Consistent inhaling of vapors can, over time, permanently damage the nervous system. Amyl nitrite has legitimate medical use re angina. Nitrites are slightly different than other inhalants as they primarily dilate blood vessels and relax the muscles (including the sphincter muscles) and thus are primarily used as sexual enhancers.

NITROUS OXIDE
(Laughing Gas, aka: N2O; NOZ)

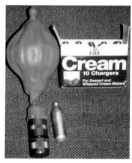

NOZ balloon with "cracker"
& cartridges

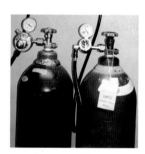

Another form of legitimate
NOZ tanks

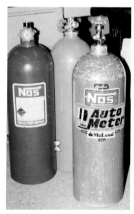

NOZ tanks from Rave

NITROUS OXIDE
(Laughing Gas aka: N2O; NOZ)

Visual Description:
Large dark blue tank (medical grade), medium size bright blue tank (vehicle/motorcycle racing performance enhancement), small metal cylinder (called "whip-its" or "whippets" –often mistaken for CO_2 but slightly shorter and dull silver in color), whipped cream dispenser (spray down for whipped cream; point upward to release the nitrous oxide propellant). May be found with a facemask (to hook via hose to large tanks), balloons (heavier grade than common balloons), or a metal or plastic "cracker" (device to release the gas into balloons from the whip-its). Nitrous Oxide is particularly popular at all-night raves.

Methods of Use:
Inhaled from balloon or tank

Duration of Effects:
Onset: Rapid
Duration: Brief

Possible Effects:
Nystagmus – Possibly
Pupils – Normal or dilated
Pulse – Elevated
Blood Pressure – Possibly lowered
Non-Convergence – Possibly
Body Temperature – Depends on Substance
Anemia (chronic use)   Dizziness
Ataxia   Euphoria (brief)
Cardiac arrhythmia   Headache
Confusion   Seizures
Disoriented   Slurred speech
Injury due to falling (brief unconsciousness common)

Overdose Symptoms:
Coma
Death

Additional Comments:
Used in dental practices, nitrous oxide is delivered with a controlled amount of oxygen. Abused from balloons, face masks, etc., the experience is quite different. Oxygen deprivation is the main issue in acute toxicity from nitrous oxide abuse.

This page intentionally left blank.

NARCOTICS

CODEINE

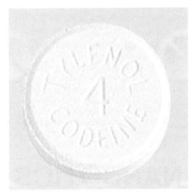

Tylenol® w/Codeine #4
(Brand name)

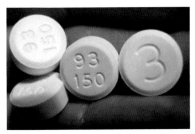

Acetaminophen w/Codeine #3
(Generic)

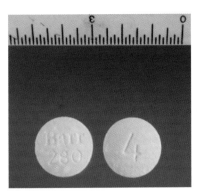

Aspirin w/Codeine #4 (Generic)

CODEINE

Trade Names & Combinations

Tylenol w/Codeine
Empirin w/Codeine
Robitussin A-C,
Prometh w/Codeine
Fiorinal (butalbital) w/Codeine

APAP w/Codeine
Codeine w/Promethazine
Phenergan w/Codeine

Visual Description:

Capsules, Dark Liquid (varying in thickness), Tablets

Methods of Use:

Ingested, Injected, Snorted

Duration of Effects:

Onset: 30-60 minutes (oral)
Peak: 1-1.5 hours (oral)
Loaded: 4-6 hours

Possible Symptoms:

Nystagmus – No
Pupils – Constricted
Pulse – Below normal
Blood Pressure – Below normal
Body Temperature – Normal/below normal
Non-Convergence – No

Depressed reflexes
Droopy eyelids (Ptosis)
Drowsiness
Dry mouth
Euphoria
Fresh puncture marks

Impaired divided attention
Low, raspy voice
Nausea
Poor muscle coordination
Profuse scratching
Vomiting

Overdose Symptoms:

Blurred vision
Cold, clammy skin
Convulsions
Constipation

Rapid, weak pulse
Slow, shallow breathing
Coma
Death

Additional Comments:

Tolerance to narcotics develops quickly, making drug dependence very likely. Phenergan w/codeine is a popular substance of abuse, popularized as "sipping syrup" in rap and hip-hop songs. The cough syrup may be consumed from a baby bottle.

FENTANYL

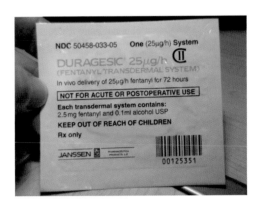

Fentanyl Patch

FENTANYL

Trade Names & Combinations

Alfenta

Actiq (lozenge lollipop)

Duragesic (patch)

Fentora (buccal tablet)

Innovar

Sublimaze

Sufenta

Legitimate Fentanyl Derivatives

Alfentanyl

Fentanyl

Lofentanyl

Sufentanyl

Illicit Analogs

Alpha-methyl fentanyl

3-methyl fentanyl

benzyl fentanyl

Visual Appearance:

White to tan powder, liquid, patch (prescription) or lollipop (lozenge on a stick) or tablet

Methods of Use:

Ingested, injected, snorted, sucked (Actiq format), or placed in mouth against gum, intended for gradual absorption (Fentora tablet format).

Duration of Effects:

Onset: Rapid w/injection (slower with patch format)

Loaded: 30 minutes to 2 hours (longer in patch format)

Possible Effects:

Nystagmus – No

Pupils – Constricted

Pulse – Below normal

Blood Pressure – Below normal

Body Temperature – Normal or below normal

Non-Convergence – No

Depressed reflexes

Droopy eyelids (Ptosis)

Drowsiness

Dry mouth

Euphoria

Vomiting

Fresh puncture marks

Impaired divided attention

Nausea

Poor muscle coordination

Profuse scratching

Overdose Symptoms:

Cold, clammy skin

Convulsions

Coma

Death

Rapid, weak pulse

Slow, shallow breathing

Additional Comments:

Prescription patches contain a concentrated gel that is being extracted and abused. Use of full amount from patch is likely to be fatal, due to the high dose (intended for transdermal, ongoing transfer, not use all at once). ***Wear gloves when handling open fentanyl patches.*** In 1979 illicit derivatives of fentanyl began appearing in the streets as "China White," a name usually associated with the very pure Southeast Asian heroin.

HEROIN
Diacetylmorphine

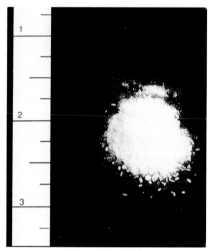

Asian-China White

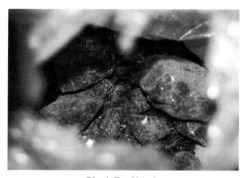

Black Tar Heroin
(Black tar-like substance has a vinegar odor)

HEROIN
Diacetylmorphine

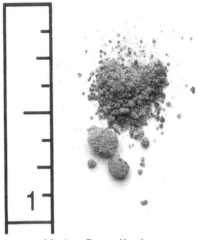

Mexican Brown Heroin
(White or Lt. Brown Powder)

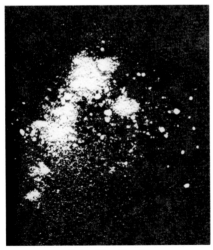

Columbian Heroin
(White powder)

HEROIN
Diacetylmorphine

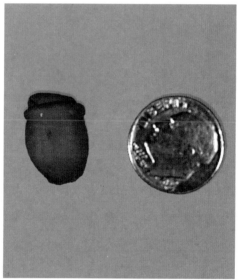

Heroin Balloon

Frequently a toy balloon is used to package Mexican Brown Powdered Heroin. The balloon is used to enable the possessor to swallow the balloon if approached by authorities. It is later retrieved after defecation.

HEROIN
Diacetylmorphine

Visual Description:
White to beige or brown powdered substance; or black tar-like substance (chunks may resemble coal, with brown powder clinging to it). May have vinegar odor.

Methods of Use:
Ingested, injected, snorted, smoked (black tar heroin)

Duration of Effects:
Onset: Rapid; varies with route of administration
Intense euphoria 45 seconds to several minutes
Peak: 1-2 hours
Loaded: 3-4 hours (Addicts may inject 2-4 times daily)

Possible Effects:
Nystagmus – No
Pupils – Constricted
Pulse – Below normal
Blood Pressure – Below normal
Body Temperature – Normal/below normal
Non-Convergence – No

Depressed reflexes
Droopy eyelids (Ptosis)
Drowsiness
Dry mouth
Euphoria
Fresh puncture marks
Impaired divided attention
Low, raspy voice
Nausea
Poor muscle coordination
Profuse scratching
Vomiting

Overdose Symptoms:
Cold, clammy skin
Coma
Convulsions
Delirium
Rapid, weak pulse
Slow, shallow breathing

Additional Comments:
Tolerance to narcotics develops quickly making drug dependence very likely.

CHEESE
(Starter Heroin)

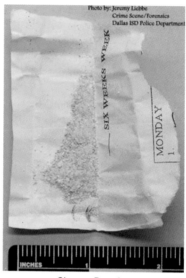

Cheese Powder

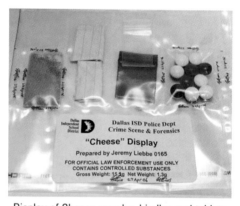

Display of Cheese powder, bindles and tablets

Photos courtesy of Ofcr. Jeremy Liebbe, Dallas Independent School District

CHEESE
(Starter Heroin)

Visual Description:

Varying shades of coarse tan powder. May be found in small paper bindles or small zip-lock baggies. "Cheese" is a mixture of heroin (usually 8 percent or less) and diphenhydramine (ground up tablets of Tylenol PM© or Benadryl©) as a way of introducing new users (typically teens) to heroin abuse.

Methods of Use:

Usually snorted through straw, tube or lower half of small ink pens

Duration of Effects:

Varies with dosage and frequency of doses
Diphenhydramine - 1 to 7 hours

Possible Effects:

Comparable to heroin
Ataxia
Drowsiness
Lethargy
Euphoria
Excessive thirst
Disorientation
Urinary retention

Withdrawal from chronic use:

Mood swings
Insomnia
Headache
Nausea/vomiting
Bone pain
Muscle spasm

Overdose Symptoms

Increased heart rate
Decreased blood pressure
Delirium
Irritability
Double vision
Coma
Respiratory depression or arrest
Death

Additional Comments:

This has been primarily a problem in the Dallas, Texas, area but there are reports Cheese has surfaced in other parts of the country. Focus has been on teens and especially Hispanic teens. Look for terms like Chees, Cheez, Chez, Chz, Queso, Keso, Kso in cell phone text messages and emails, for example.

HYDROMORPHONE
Dilaudid

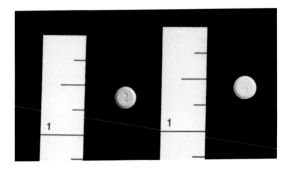

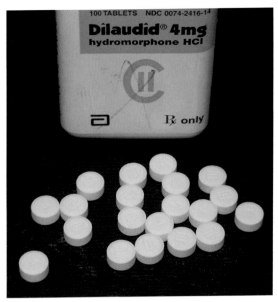

Dilaudid 4mg Tablets

HYDROMORPHONE
Dilaudid

Visual Description:
Powder, pills (white, pink, orange, light green, yellow)
1 - 8 mg.

Methods of Use:
Ingested, Injected or Snorted

Duration of Effects:
Onset: 15-30 minutes
Peak: 30-60 minutes
Duration: 4-6 Hours

Possible Effects:
Nystagmus – No
Pupils – Constricted
Pulse – Below normal
Blood Pressure – Below Normal
Body Temperature – Normal/below normal
Non-Convergence – No
Depressed reflexes
Droopy eyelids (Ptosis)
Drowsiness
Dry mouth
Euphoria
Fresh puncture marks
Impaired divided attention
Low, raspy voice
Nausea
Poor muscle coordination
Profuse scratching
Vomiting

Overdose Symptoms:

Cold, clammy skin	Slow, shallow breathing
Convulsions	Rapid, weak pulse
Coma	Death

Additional Comments:
Tolerance to narcotics develops quickly, making drug dependence very likely.

HYDROCODONE

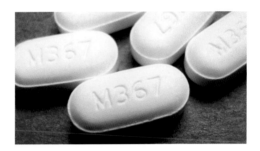

APAP / Hydrocodone

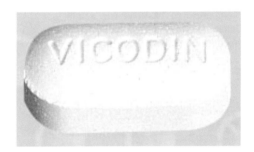

Vicodin (front)

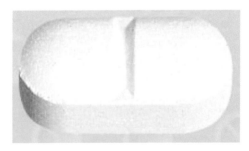

Vicodin (back)

HYDROCODONE

Trade Names & Combinations

Hydrocodone & Acetaminophen - Vicodin, Lorcet, Lortab, Norco

Tussionex - cough syrup

Hydrocodone & Aspirin -Damason

Hydrocodone & Homatropine - Hycodan

Hydrocodone & Ibuprofen - Vicoprofen

Visual Description:

Liquid, pills (oblong pills in white, light pink, bright pink, orange, yellow, light blue or red capsules), powder

Methods of Use:

Ingested, injected, snorted

Duration of Effects:

Loaded: 4-8 hours

Possible Effects:

Nystagmus – No

Pupils – Constricted

Pulse – Below normal

Blood Pressure – Below normal

Body Temperature – Normal or below normal

Non-Convergence – No

Depressed reflexes

Droopy eyelids (Ptosis)

Drowsiness

Dry mouth

Euphoria

Fresh puncture marks

Impaired divided attention

Low, raspy voice

Nausea

Poor muscle coordination

Profuse scratching

Vomiting

Overdose Symptoms:

Cold, clammy skin	Rapid, weak pulse
Convulsions	Slow, shallow breathing
Coma	Death

Additional Comments:

Tolerance to narcotics develops very quickly, making drug dependence very likely.

MEPERIDINE

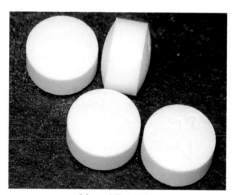

Meperidine Tabs

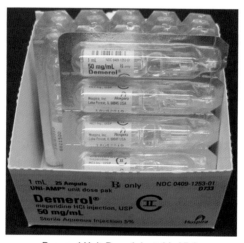

Demerol Unit Dose Injectable Vials

MEPERIDINE

Trade Names & Combinations
Demerol
Meperitab

Visual Description:
Tablets (white, 50-100 mg), Clear Liquid, White Powder

Methods of Use:
Ingested, Injected, Snorted

Duration of Effects:
Onset: 10-15 minutes
Peak: 1 hour
Duration: 2-6 Hours

Possible Symptoms:
Nystagmus – No
Pupils – Constricted
Pulse – Below normal
Blood Pressure – Below normal
Body Temperature – Normal/Below normal
Non-Convergence – No
Depressed reflexes
Droopy eyelids (Ptosis)
Drowsiness
Dry mouth
Euphoria
Fresh puncture marks
Impaired divided attention
Low, raspy voice
Nausea
Poor muscle coordination
Profuse scratching
Vomiting

Overdose Symptoms:
Cold, clammy skin
Convulsions
Rapid, weak pulse
Slow, Shallow Breathing
Coma
Death

Additional Comments:
Tolerance to narcotics develops quickly, making drug dependence very likely.

METHADONE
(Aka: Dolophine, Methadose)

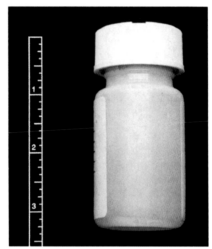

Methadone Liquid

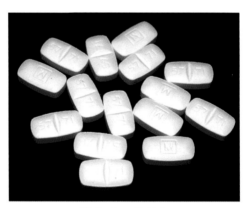

Methadone Tablets

METHADONE
(Aka: Dolophine, Methadose)

Trade Names
> Dolophine
> Methadose
> Metadol (Canadian)

Visual Description:
> Clear, pink liquid or white or peach tablet, 5-40 mg

Methods of Use:
> Ingested, Injected, Snorted

Duration of Effects:
> Onset: 30-60 minutes
> Duration: 4-8 Hours (w/repeated doses, increased to 22-24 hrs

Possible Effects:
> **Nystagmus** – No
> **Pupils** – Possibly constricted
> **Pulse** – Below normal
> **Blood Pressure** – Below normal
> **Body Temperature** – Normal/below normal
> **Non-Convergence** – No

> Depressed reflexes
> Droopy eyelids (Ptosis)
> Drowsiness
> Dry mouth
> Euphoria
> Fresh puncture marks
> Impaired divided attention
> Low, raspy voice
> Nausea
> Poor motor coordination
> Vomiting

Overdose Symptoms:
> Cold, clammy skin
> Convulsions
> Coma
> Rapid, weak pulse
> Slow, shallow breathing
> Death

Additional Comments:
> When taken in proper doses, methadone should not show any effects. It is used to keep the heroin addict "well" and reduce the craving for heroin. They remain addicted to the opioid, but methadone blocks the high from heroin and does not provide a euphoric rush. It is only effective in cases of addiction to heroin, morphine, and other opioid drugs; it is not an effective treatment for other drugs of abuse. Law enforcement officers are typically familiar only with the use of methadone in heroin addiction treatment. In fact, it is also a pain medication being increasingly widely used by doctors to treat pain and thus even more widely abused. Methadone stays in the system a long time, meaning it can build up and can reach toxic levels. Deaths from methadone overdose have been increasing.

MORPHINE

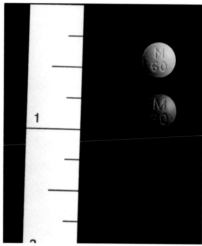

Morphine Tablets

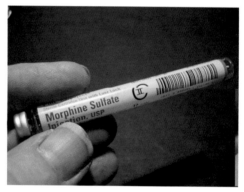

Morphine Injectable

MORPHINE

Trade Names
MS Contin
Avinza
Roxanol
Duramorph

Visual Description:
Tablets, Pink Liquid

Methods of Use:
Ingested, Injected, Snorted

Duration of Effects:
Onset: Rapid w/injection; 15-60 minutes oral
Peak: 50-90 minutes; 15-60 minutes injected
Impaired: 3-6 Hours

Possible Effects:
Nystagmus – No
Pupils – Constricted
Pulse – Below normal
Blood Pressure – Below normal
Body Temperature – Normal/below normal
Non-Convergence – No

Depressed reflexes	Impaired divided attention
Droopy eyelids (Ptosis)	Low, raspy voice
Drowsiness	Nausea
Dry mouth	Poor motor coordination
Euphoria	Profuse scratching
Fresh puncture marks	Vomiting

Overdose Symptoms:
Cold, clammy skin
Convulsions
Rapid, weak pulse
Slow, shallow breathing
Coma
Death

Additional Comments:
Tolerance to narcotics develops quickly making drug dependence very likely.

OPIUM

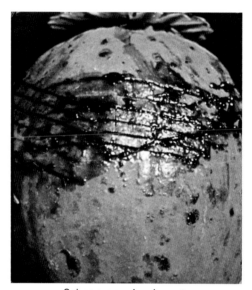

Opium poppy showing cuts
to extract the raw opium.

OPIUM

Visual Description:
Dark Brown Chunks, Powder

Methods of Use:
Injected, Ingested (liquid, tea), Smoked, Snorted

Duration of Effects:
Impaired: 4-6 Hours

Possible Effects:
Nystagmus – No
Pupils – Constricted
Pulse – Below normal
Blood Pressure – Below normal
Body Temperature – Normal/below normal
Non-Convergence – No

Depressed reflexes
Droopy eyelids (Ptosis)
Drowsiness
Dry mouth
Euphoria
Fresh puncture marks
Impaired divided attention
Low, raspy voice
Nausea
Poor motor coordination
Profuse scratching
Vomiting

Overdose Symptoms:
Apnea
Cold, clammy skin
Convulsions
Delirium
Pulmonary edema
Rapid, weak pulse
Slow, shallow breathing
Coma
Death

Additional Comments:
Tolerance to narcotics develops quickly making drug dependence very likely.

OXYCODONE

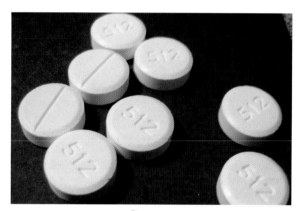

Percocet

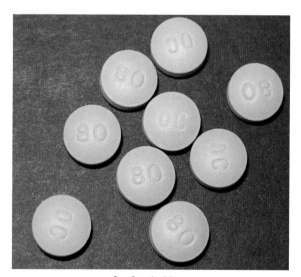

OxyContin 80mg

OXYCODONE

Common Trade Names & Combinations
  Oxycodone - OxyContin, Oxydose, OxyFast, Tylox
  Oxycodone & Acetaminophen - Percocet, Roxicet, Endocet,
    Oxycocet (Canadian)
  Oxycodone & Aspirin - Percodan, Endodan,
    Oxycodan (Canadian)

Visual Description
  Tablets, Drops, Liquid

Methods of Use
  Ingested, Injected, Snorted

Duration of Effects
  Onset: 15-30 minutes (oral)
  Impaired: 4-6 Hours

Possible Effects
  Nystagmus – No
  Pupils – Constricted
  Pulse – Below normal
  Blood Pressure – Below normal
  Body Temperature – Normal/below normal
  Non-Convergence – No

Depressed reflexes	Impaired divided attention
Droopy eyelids (Ptosis)	Low, raspy voice
Drowsiness	Nausea
Dry mouth	Poor motor coordination
Euphoria	Profuse scratching
Fresh puncture marks	Vomiting

Overdose Symptoms:
  Cold, clammy skin
  Convulsions
  Rapid, weak pulse
  Slow, shallow breathing
  Coma
  Death

Additional Comments:
  Tolerance to narcotics develops quickly making drug dependence very likely.

ADDITIONAL NARCOTICS

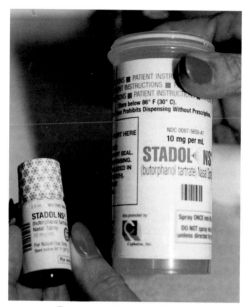

Butorphanol Tartrate - Stadol

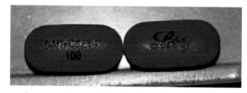

Propoxyphene & Acetaminophen - Darvocet

ADDITIONAL NARCOTICS

Drug – Trade names (representative)
> **Buprenorphine** -Buprenex, Subutex 7-24 hours duration
> **Butorphanol Tartrate** - Stadol (nasal spray) 3-6 hours duration
> **Propoxyphene & Acetaminophen** - Darvocet 4-6 hours duration
> **Propoxyphene** - Darvon, Darvon-N 4-6 hours duration
> **Nalbuphine** - Nubain 3-6 hours duration
> **Pentazocine** - Talwin, Talacen, Talwin NX 2-3 hours duration
> **Tramadol** - Ultram 6-8 hours duration

Additional Comments:
> Effects generally similar to other narcotic analgesics

KRATOM
Botanical Name: Mitragyna speciosa

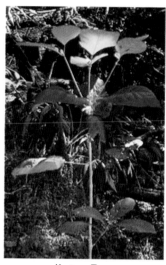

Kratom Tree

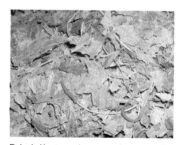

Dried Kratom leaves about to be brewed into a euphoric tea.

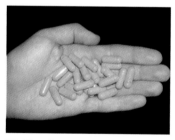

25 Size 0 capsules of 500mg of Kratom. It takes approximately 10 caps to induce an opiate-like euphoria.

KRATOM
Botanical Name: Mitragyna speciosa

Visual Description:

Source is a tropical tree primarily in South East Asia, up to 50 feet tall; same family as coffee tree. Distributed as leaves (whole or crushed), powder, extract, resin extract "pies" or pellets. Seeds also seen available on Internet

Methods of Use:

Leaf is chewed for stimulant effect or brewed into tea. May also be boiled & mixed with cola or cough syrup. Some reports of "juice" preparation. Described as having a combination of stimulant and opiate effects, usually varying with dosage.

Duration of Effects:

Onset within 10 minutes, reportedly fading within several hours

Possible Effects:

Low doses may produce primarily stimulant effects
>   Increased alertness
>   Talkativeness
>   Increased physical activity

Higher doses produce opiate effects
>   Reduced pain response
>   Sedation
>   Mild euphoria

Addiction may result from chronic use
Psychoactive effects may result especially with chronic use
>   Hallucinations
>   Confusion

Constipation
Nausea

Street Names:

Thang, Kakuam, Thom, Ketum

Additional Comments:

Kratom is unscheduled in the U.S. at this time. Knowledge of this drug is somewhat limited. Some have reported using it to mitigate the withdrawal from opiates. It is an unusual drug with varying effects. We are including it in the NARCOTICS section at this time due to its primary effects being most comparable to opiates.

This page intentionally left blank.

DISSOCIATIVE ANESTHETICS

PCP
Phencyclidine

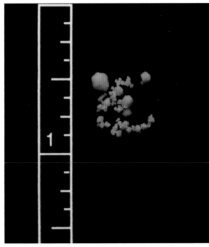

Powdered PCP

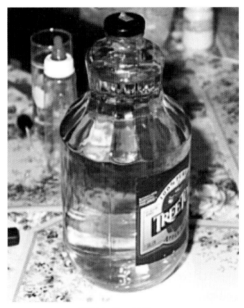

PCP in Liquid Form

PCP
Phencyclidine

Visual Description:
White or brown powder, pills, capsules, light to medium gold liquid. Occasionally found mixed with meth in pills sold as Ecstasy

Methods of Use:
Ingested; smoked (marijuana or tobacco cigarette dipped in PCP); absorbed; inhaled; injected.

Duration of Effects:
Onset: 1-5 Minutes   Loaded: 4-6 Hours
Peak: 15-30 Minutes
Overdose Effects: 24 Hrs or Longer

Possible Effects:
Nystagmus – Yes (Vertical & Horizontal)
Pupils – Near normal
Pulse – Elevated
Blood Pressure – Elevated
Body Temperature – Elevated
Non-Convergence – Yes

Agitation & aggressive	Long, intense trips
Analgesia (pain block, high pain threshold)	Muscle rigidity
Catatonia	Non-communicative
Cyclic behavior	Odor of substance
Disoriented	Paranoia
Dysphoria	Perspiring
Eyelid tremors	Repetitive speech
Emergence delirium	Synesthesia
Fearful	Warm to the touch
Fascination w/water	

Overdose Symptoms:
Bizarre behavior
Long, intense trips
Psychosis
Violence
Death

Additional Comments:
"Embalming fluid" is an old nickname for PCP. Formaldehyde (embalming fluid ingredient) was often added to slow the burn. More recently, some have abused so-called wet, fry or illy sticks which are marijuana cigarettes dipped in either pure PCP, the combination, or pure formaldehyde (produces bizarre behavior but not the pain blocking effect of PCP). Avoid loud noises, bright lights or sudden movements with subjects under the influence.

KETAMINE
(Special K)

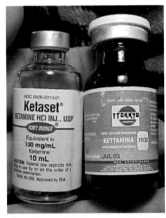

Legitimate (left) and counterfeit
(right) Ketamine vials

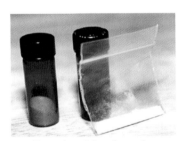

Ketamine vial and powder

KETAMINE
(Special K)

Visual Description:
Clear liquid (very light amber color) often in injectable-type vial; white powder.

Methods of Use:
Ingested; snorted; smoked; injected; rectal insertion.

Duration of Effects:
Onset: Rapid
Pain Block: 30 minutes to 2 hours (dose dependent)
Amnesia effect up to 2 hours

Possible Effects:
Nystagmus – yes
Pupils – Near normal
Pulse – Elevated
Blood Pressure – Elevated
Body Temperature – Elevated
Non-Convergence – Yes
Analgesia (pain block)
Apnea
Catatonic state (The K-Hole)
Delirium
Emergence delirium (bizarre or violent behavior)
Flashbacks
Hallucinations (vivid)
Insomnia
Seizures
Tremors
Vomiting
Coma
Cardiac arrest

Additional Comments:
Avoid stimulation such as loud noises and rapid movements around subjects under the influence to reduce emergence delirium. May have flashbacks.

DEXTROMETHORPHAN
(DXM)
Cough Suppressant

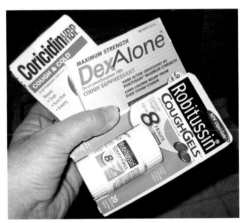

Common commercial DXM products

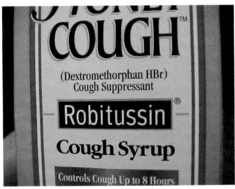

Common liquid DXM product

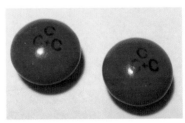

DXM – Street name "Triple C" tablets

DEXTROMETHORPHAN
(DXM)
Cough Suppressant

DXM is a common ingredient as a cough suppressant in numerous over-the-counter products and is not a controlled substance at this time. It is a highly abused substance nationwide, especially among young teens because of its legal availability. Even teens with money to buy the product sometimes shoplift because this act is virtually part of the culture of the DXM crowd. Normal dosing involves one or two pills or doses of cough syrup every four hours. Abusers may take 10 to 45 pills at a time or fairly rapid succession as they seek to achieve the various "plateaus" of experiences described on Internet websites such as www.dextroverse.org and www.erowid.org, two of many pro-drug websites. Some rank DXM with depressants but in higher doses, it is closer in effects to PCP and ketamine, making it an atypical dissociative anesthetic or narcotic analgesic. The effects are also complicated by the fact that it is often taken in pills with other ingredients as well, causing variations on effect. Websites instruct abusers on extracting DXM from cough syrups and pills that contain other medications to avoid the interactions and high doses of the other ingredients.

Duration:
Onset: 15-30 minutes (oral), more rapid if snorted
Duration 6 hours

Visual Description:
Gel capsule, pill or liquid, varying with product, and may be seen in powder form.

Possible Effects:

Excitation	Hypertension
Respiratory depression	Hyperthermia
Insomnia	Ataxia
Coma	Tremors
Fever	Hyperactivity, and in high doses dissociative effects similar to PCP or ketamine

Terms & Products:
Robotripping, Robitussin DM, Coricidin Cough & Cold (aka: CCC, Triple C), The Matrix (for the red CCC pills), Skittles and Skittling, DexAlone, Simply Cough, Vicks 44 Cough Relief, Benylin, Creomulsion Cough, ElixSure, Silphen DMetc. Any product containing DXM is a potential target for abuse. DexAlone contains no other ingredients.

DISSOCIATIVE ANESTHETICS

This page intentionally left blank.

STIMULANTS

AMPHETAMINES

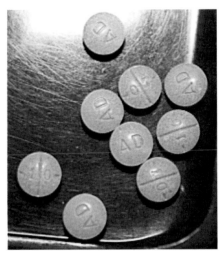

Amphetamine & Dextroamphetamine
Adderall 10 mg

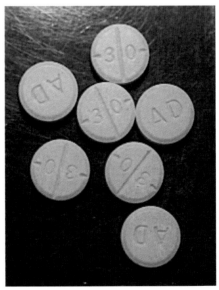

Amphetamine & Dextroamphetamine
Adderall 30 mg

AMPHETAMINES

Drug Name – Representative Tradename
  Amphetamine and Dextroamphetamine – Adderall
  Dextroamphetamine – Dexedrine, Dextrostat (Canada)
  Methylphenidate – Ritalin, Concerta, Metadate,
                          Riphenidate (Canada)
  Pemoline – Cylert (no longer marketed in the U.S.)
  Methamphetamine – Desoxyn

Visual Description:
  Various shapes/colors/doses of capsules or pills, depending on brand and dosage. May also be found in powder.

Methods of Use:
  These are prescription drugs typically used for treatment of attention deficit disorders, narcolepsy or exogenous obesity. But they have become widely diverted as stay-awake pills for students, working adults, etc. Abusers may take them as pills or crush them into powder for snorting or even convert to liquid for injecting.

Duration of Effects:
  Onset: 30 seconds (snorted/injected) to 1½ hours (oral)
  Duration: 4-8 hours (Concerta is a slow-release version of Ritalin)

Possible Effects:

Nystagmus – No	**Blood Pressure** – Elevated
Pupils – Dilated	**Body Temperature** – Elevated
Pulse – Elevated	**Non-Convergence** – No
Anxiety	Headaches
Arrhythmia	Hypertension
Body tremors	Impaired divided attention
Decreased appetite	Increased alertness
Dizziness	Insomnia
Dry mouth	Restlessness
Euphoria	Sexual impairment
Excitation	Sweating
Grinding teeth (bruxism)	Weight loss
Psychomotor agitation or retardation	Hallucinations

Overdose Symptoms:

Convulsions	Vomiting
Coma	Seizures
Death	

Additional Comments:
  High levels of amphetamines or injected doses can create a sudden rise in blood pressure that can cause a stroke, very high fever or heart attack. Prolonged use can cause hallucination, delusions and paranoia. Even chewing tablets versus swallowing can increase side effects and decrease efficacy for those using legitimately. Pemoline dropped due to increased liver function risks.

COCAINE
(Crack or Freebase)

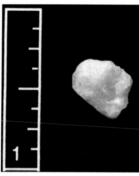

Cocaine - Crack or Freebase

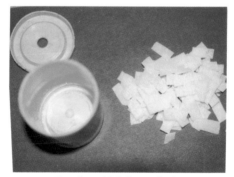

Cocaine - 18th Street Style

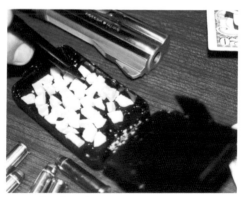

Cocaine - Dope, Money and the Gun

COCAINE
(Crack or Freebase)

Visual Description:
Light brown, beige or white crystalline rocks often packaged in small vials or zip-lock plastic bags. May also be found in "cookie" shapes when made in the bottom of small containers and not yet broken/cut into pieces. Though most often made with baking soda, coke powder may also be converted with baking soda, flour, yeast and carbonated beverage, resulting in a more bubbled texture.

Methods of Use:
Smoked

Duration of Effects:
Onset: 8-30 seconds   Duration: 10-20 minutes
Peak: 5 minutes

Possible Effects:
Nystagmus – No
Pupils – Dilated
Pulse – Elevated
Blood Pressure – Elevated
Body Temperature – Elevated
Non Convergence – No

Anxiety	Hallucinations
Apnea	Hypertension
Ataxia	Impaired divided attention
Body tremors	Impotence
Decreased appetite	Increased alertness
Dental erosion (chronic use)	Insomnia
Depression	Paranoia
Dizziness	Restlessness
Dry mouth	Running/red/bleeding nose
Euphoria	Seizures
Excitation	Sweating
Fresh puncture marks	Talkative
Grinding teeth (bruxism)	Weight loss
Headaches	

Overdose Symptoms:

Agitation, extreme	Coma
Convulsions	Death

Additional Comments:
The 18th Street Gang is known for its signature "wafer" rock cocaine, shaped in thin squares or rectangles resembling wafers or pasta, rather than the traditional "rock" shapes. Traditional rock cocaine somewhat resembles pieces of macadamia nut, though harder in texture. Freebasing cocaine using ether is a less common and much more dangerous method (severe burns can result if smoked before the ether has completely evaporated). Waxy or soapy in appearance.

COCAINE

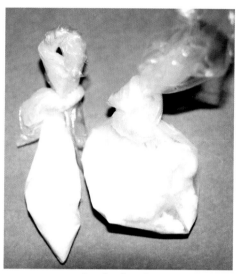

Cocaine Powder

Powdered Cocaine is placed on a mirror or piece of glass or other flat, non-porous surface. It is then chopped into a fine powder with a razor blade or credit card. The Cocaine is then spread into thin lines, and the lines are then snorted through a tube, drinking straw or rolled currency. See page 138.

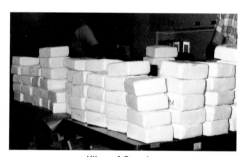

Kilos of Cocaine

COCAINE

Visual Description:
White crystalline (shiny) powder (may be "cut" or diluted with other products such as procaine, lidocaine, mannitol, ephedrine, sucrose, lactose, tetracaine, benzocaine, etc., to extend the quantity of product). Has surfaced as "black" cocaine to attempt to fool law enforcement, using charcoal, cobalt, iron dust, etc., to alter the color. May be found in bindles, plastic baggies, or pressed into kilos. Markings on kilos may indicate the producer or the intended recipient.

Methods of Use:
Snorted, Injected. (Chewing coca leaf provides a mild stimulant effect).

Duration of Effects:
Onset

	Injected: immediate	Snorted: 2-3 minutes
	Oral: within 1 hour	

Loaded:
5-45 minutes   Oral ingestion: 1-2 hours
                                          Peak: 5-15 minutes

Possible Effects:

Nystagmus – No   **Pupils** – Dilated
Pulse – Elevated   **Blood Pressure** – Elevated
Body Temperature – Elevated
Non-Convergence – No

Anxiety	Hallucinations
Apnea	Hypertension
Ataxia	Impotence
Body tremors	Impaired divided attention
Decreased appetite	Increased alertness
Dental erosion (chronic use)	Insomnia
Depression	Paranoia
Dizziness	Restlessness
Dry mouth	Running/red/bleeding nose
Euphoria	Seizures
Excitation	Sweating
Fresh puncture marks	Talkative
Grinding teeth (bruxism)	Weight loss
Headaches	

Overdose Symptoms:

Agitation, extreme	Convulsions
Coma	Death

Additional Comments:
Occasional use of cocaine can cause an irritated, stuffy or blood nose, while long-term use may result in ulceration of the mucous membranes of the nose or complete perforation of the nasal septum. Schedule II because it does have limited legitimate use as a topical anesthesia of the mucous membranes for medical procedures.

METHAMPHETAMINE
(Crank or Speed)

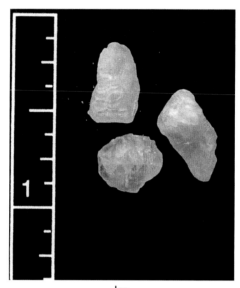

Ice

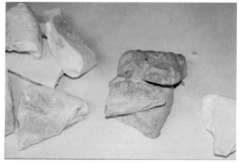

Varied Colors of Methamphetamine

METHAMPHETAMINE
(Crank or Speed)

Visual Description:
Powder or chunks of various shades from white to beige, orange or pink (dye from type of source pills used for ephedrine or pseudoephedrine). Like cocaine, it may be adulterated with "cuts" to extend the quantity or to clean up the color; common cut is a dietary supplement MSM (methyl-sulfonyl methane). Also marketed in prescription tablet as Desoxyn for short-term weight loss and attention deficit disorder.

"Ice" or crystal meth: white crystalline rock; freebase form of methamphetamine, typically of high purity. May look like chunks of ice or shards of glass.

Methods of Use:
Injected, smoked, snorted, swallowed

Duration of Effects:
Onset: 5-20 minutes (snorted) 30-60 minutes (oral) within seconds (smoked)
Duration: 6-18 hours

Possible Effects:

Nystagmus – No	**Blood Pressure** – Elevated
Pupils – Dilated	**Body Temperature** – Elevated
Pulse – Elevated	**Non-Convergence** – No
Anxiety	Increased alertness
Body tremors	Insomnia
Decreased appetite	Loss of coordination
Dizziness	Paranoia
Dry mouth	Puncture marks
Euphoria	Restlessness
Excitation	Sexual stimulation
Grinding teeth (bruxism)	Sweating
Hallucinations	Weight loss
Impaired divided attention	

Overdose Symptoms:

Agitation	Hallucinations
Coma	Psychosis
Convulsions	Death

Additional Comments:
Methamphetamine can be made in a variety of ways, depending on the quantity being made and the materials available. Large meth labs may involve extensive chemical lists and laboratory equipment; small labs may involve only easily obtained ingredients and homemade conversion of common items. "Ice" is crystal meth, a smokable form of methamphetamine. Use first started in the Far East, then Hawaii, with use/manufacturing based in South Korea, the Philippines, Honk Kong and Japan. Now found in a much more widespread pattern in the U.S.

METHCATHINONE
N-Methyl-Cathinone (aka: "Cat")

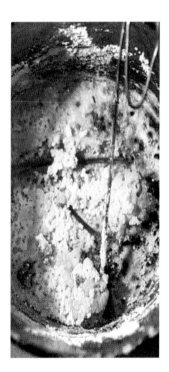
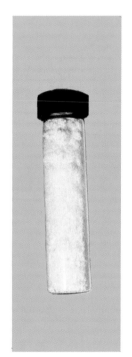

METHCATHINONE
N-Methyl-Cathinone (aka: "Cat")

Visual Description:
Off-white, light yellow or beige powder

Methods of Use:
Injected, snorted, smoked or taken orally

Duration of Effects:
Loaded from 30 minutes to 24 hours depending on dosage

Possible Effects:
Nystagmus – No
Pupils – Dilated
Pulse – Elevated
Blood Pressure – Elevated
Body Temperature – Elevated
Non-Convergence – No

Anxiety	Impaired divided attention
Body tremors	Increased alertness
Decreased appetite	Insomnia
Dizziness	Loss of coordination
Euphoria	Paranoia
Excitation	Puncture marks
Grinding teeth (bruxism)	Restlessness
Hallucinations	

Overdose Symptoms:

Agitation	Psychosis
Convulsions	Coma
Fever	Death
Hallucinations	

Additional Comments:
Though easily made and similar to methamphetamine, this drug has been mostly centered in the Midwest and not widely favored. Just as with methamphetamine, ephedrine or pseudoephedrine is the key ingredient. Norephedrine (phenylpropanolamine) can be substituted, resulting in cathinone rather than methcathinone (see Cathinone).

In early 2009 a drug believed to be 4-methylmethcathinone (4-MMC) (aka: "Sunshine") surfaced in Oregon. This drug had been reported earlier in Australia, Sweden and Denmark. Though related chemically to methcathinone, the effects of methylmethcathinone are supposedly akin to crystal meth plus some of the psychotropic effects of MDMA (Ecstasy) and other phenethylamines. By late 2009 it was growing across the international club scene and is often referred to as MEPHEDRONE (not to be confused with methedrone, methadone, or other drugs with similar names). This is a stimulant often marketed on the Internet as "plant food." It has now surfaced across the U.S. It has been banned in Sweden, due to a death there, and some other countries. It is also known as drone, bubble or bubbles, meow meow, MM-Cat or M-Cat.

CATHINONE
Aka: Khat – Catha Edulis plant
(Pronounced "Cot")

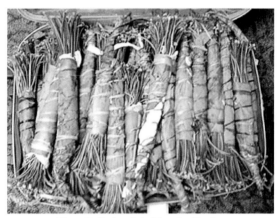

Khat - Rolled and tied for distribution

CATHINONE
Aka: Khat – Catha Edulis plant
(Pronounced "Cot")

Visual Description:
White powder if synthesized (similar to making methamphetamine or methcathinone). Or, plant material from a flowering evergreen tree or large shrub. Leaves are described as green to crimson-brown and glossy, but may become yellow-green and leathery as they age/dry.

Methods of Use:
Chewing the leaves, drinking plant juice

Duration of Effects:
Onset: 20 minutes   Duration: 2 hours

Possible Effects:
Nystagmus – No
Pupils – Dilated
Pulse – Elevated
Blood Pressure – Elevated
Body Temperature – Elevated
Non-Convergence – No

Anesthetic properties	Excitation
Anxiety	Impaired divided attention
Body tremors	Increased alertness
Decreased appetite	Insomnia
Dizziness	Paranoia
Euphoria	Restlessness

Overdose Symptoms:
Breathing difficulties
Convulsions
Psychosis
Coma
Death

Additional Comments:
Plant comes primarily from Eastern Africa at high altitudes. Khat contains cathinone when leaves are fresh. As leaves dry (unrefrigerated more than 48 hours), contents deteriorate to contain only cathine, a lesser stimulant.

ADDITIONAL STIMULANTS

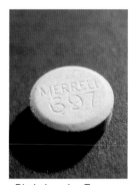

Diethylpropion Tenuate

Courtesy of Christine Larson, AZDPS

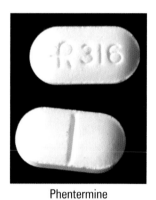

Phentermine

Courtesy of Christine Larson, AZDPS

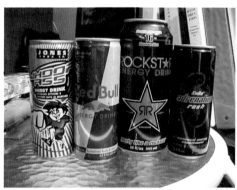

Drinks Containing Taurine

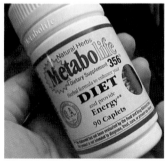

Caplet contains 12mg ephedrine group alkaloids

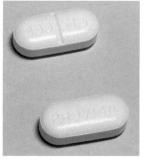

Provigil 200mg

ADDITIONAL STIMULANTS

Drug Name – Representative Tradename
>   **Diethylpropion** – Tenuate, Dospan (anorectic - for weight loss, stimulant effects)
>   **Mazindol** – Mazanor, Sanorex (anorectic for weight loss and narcolepsy)
>   **Phenmetrazine** – Nistenal, Preludin (anorectic)
>   **Phendimetrazine** – Prelu-2 (anorectic)
>   **Benzphetamine** – Didrex (anorectic)
>   **Phentermine** – Adipex, Fastin, Ionamin (anorectic)
>   **Fenfluramine** or **Dexfenfluramine** – Pondimin, Redux

Visual Description:
>   Various pills, capsules or powder

Methods of Use:
>   Taken as pills or snorted

Duration of Effects:
>   Similar to other stimulants, varying with product

Possible Effects:
>   Similar to other stimulants

Additional Comments:
>   Fen Phen, a once popular diet pill combination, was a combination of phentermine and fenfluramine or dexfenfluramine that was linked to excessive cases of primary pulmonary hypertension, resulting in numerous lawsuits.

OTHER CHEMICALS WITH STIMULANT PROPERTIES

Ephedrine & Pseudoephedrine (also Ma Huang)
Bitter Orange - citrus aurantium (synephrine)
Kola nut extract
Taurine (featured in large quantity in numerous energy drinks)
Caffeine (also called Guarana)
Yohimbe

Additional Comments:
>   These chemicals may cause typical stimulant properties such as increased heart rate, increased body temperature, etc., and may be encountered in DUI or overdose cases. Bitter orange, kola nut, taurine and caffeine are often included in supplements in very large quantities as ephedrine alternatives or in addition to ephedrine, but may harbor some of the same risk factors as taking ephedrine. Relatively little research has been done re ongoing ingestion of large quantities of such ingredients.

(cont'd next pg.)

ADDITIONAL EMERGING STIMULANTS OF ABUSE

Modafinil – Provigil (daytime sleepiness, narcolepsy)

Modafinil is said to be relatively free of typical stimulant side effects such as agitation, irritability, nervousness, euphoria or the potential for paranoid delusion and addiction that are common to other stimulants (when used a directed). Modafinil targets very specific regions of the brain believed to regulate normal wakefulness. This drug is being touted for shift-work related sleepiness, daytime sleepiness and narcolepsy. While "abuse" may not follow traditional stimulant patterns, over use of it may result in fatigue after the fact and thus result in impaired driving. Effects may include blurred vision, dizziness, dry mouth, insomnia, depression, confusion, mood swings, nervousness, anxiety or agitation, etc.

Fenethylline — Captagon & Theophylline – Slo-Phyllin

Captagon is an internationally recognized trademark name for the drug fenethylline; it is no longer legally made and is not used in the U.S. under any trademark. Slo-Phyllin is a U.S. trademark name for the drug theophylline, which is used for respiratory diseases, such as asthma. Fenethylline metabolizes (breaks down) in the human body into amphetamine and theophylline (which is a lower level stimulant, somewhat similar to caffeine). Though no longer legally made, fenethylline is still commonly referred to as Captagon and is an increasingly popular drug of abuse in the Arab countries, particularly Saudi Arabia. Large seizures are becoming common in that region. Pills may resemble MDMA (Ecstasy) and may even be sold as Ecstasy. Contents may actually be illegally-made fenethylline or other mixtures merely being represented as fenethylline. Due to the international trafficking patterns of Ecstasy- type drugs and the increased contact of American troops, contractors and others with countries abusing fenethylline, there is a potential for growing exposure in the U.S. to fenethylline and a potential for increased abuse interest in the caffeine-level stimulant theophylline.

ANDROGENIC ANABOLIC STEROIDS

ANDROGENIC ANABOLIC STEROIDS

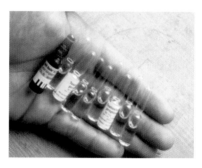

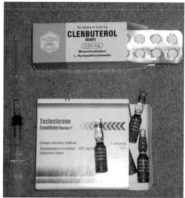

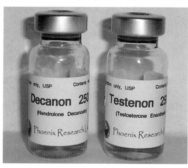

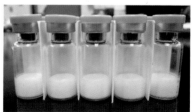

Photo courtesy South Dakota Highway Patrol

ANDROGENIC ANABOLIC STEROIDS

Street Names:
   Juice, roids, stackers, gym candy, pumpers, arnolds

Representative names:
   Anadrol (oxymetholone)
   Dianabol (methandrostenolone)
   Deca-Durabolin (nandrolone decanoate)
   Depo-Testosterone (testosterone cypionate)
   Durabolin (nandrolone phenpropionate)
   Equipose (veterinary product, boldenone undecylenate)
   Halotestin (fluoxymesterone)
   Oxandrin (oxandrolone)
   Winstrol (stanozolol)

Visual Description:
   Various shapes and colors of pills, clear or yellow to gold colored
   liquid in glass vials, loaded syringes

Methods of Use:
   Taken orally or most commonly injected (often in unusual
   locations, trying to avoid areas visual when wearing swim trunks
   or bikini). Multiple doses of various anabolic steroids (stacking)
   is typically done to maximize effectiveness in case some of the
   product is fake and worthless. Typically taken for a specific
   period, followed by a period off of them and then resuming use
   (called "cycling"). Legitimate steroids also include gels or
   patches or implanted pellets. Abuse levels may be up to 100
   times the therapeutic amounts.

General Effects:

Liver disorders (jaundice, liver damage)	Cholesterol changes
Cancer risks	Infertility
Adverse cardiovascular effects	Severe acne
Fluid retention	High blood pressure
Increased aggression or bizarre behavior (known as "roid rage")	

Other Effects - Teens:
   Prematurely stunted skeletal growth
   Rapid rate of puberty changes

Other Effects - Males:
   Atrophy of testicles
   Reduced sperm production
   Baldness
   Development of breasts (gynecomastia, also called "bitch tits")
   Increased chance of prostate enlargement and/or cancer

Other Effects - Females:

Facial hair growth	Male-pattern baldness
Enlarged clitoris	Menstrual irregularity
Masculinization of facial hair, depth of voice	

(cont'd next pg.)

ANDROGENIC ANABOLIC STEROIDS

Additional Comments:

Legally used for body wasting diseases (patients with AIDS, for example) and those born with insufficient natural production of testosterone for normal development. Abused illegally by athletes (and some law enforcement officers & firefighters) for increased strength and size, by bodybuilders for dramatic body appearance and by teens for athletic performance, size (often to overcome being victim of bullying) or appearance (females, for example, seeking lean look by taking steroids but not doing intense workouts which would build bulk).

PARAPHERNALIA IDENTIFICATION AND DESCRIPTIONS

MARIJUANA SMOKING PARAPHERNALIA

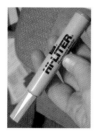
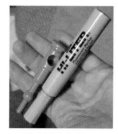
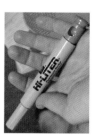

HI-LITER® Pipe

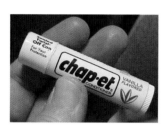
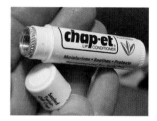

"Chapstick" Pipe

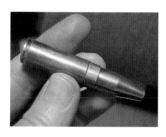
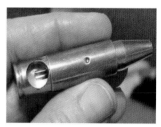

Bullet Pipe

MARIJUANA ROACH CLIPS

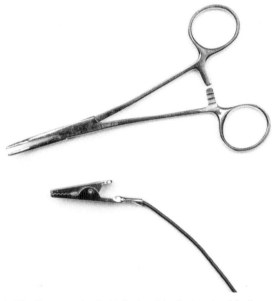

"Roach Clips" are used to hold the last bit of a burning Marijuana cigarette. In addition to the devices shown, small tweezers may also be used.

OTHER TYPES OF SMOKING
PARAPHERNALIA

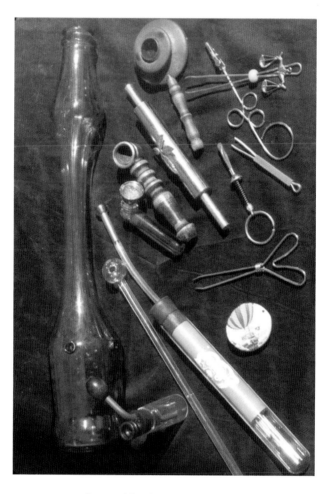

Assorted Crack, Hash & Marijuana
Smoking Paraphernalia

FREEBASE SMOKING PIPE

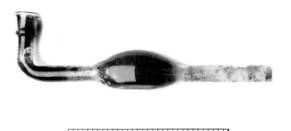

After placing a piece of copper scouring pad, steel wool or Brillo Pad in the bowl, the Freebase Rock is placed on top and lit. The rock will begin to vaporize and melt. Since the vapors are heavier than air, they drop into the neck of the pipe and are drawn into the lungs. Some pipes have a bulge or chamber in the neck of the pipe that is used to collect the vapor and allow it to accumulate before it is inhaled into the lungs. This chamber is also used for cooling the vapor. A glass or metal tube, called a **"Straight Shooter"** is also used. Often made from automotive radio antennas, they are readily obtained and can be easily dropped if authorities should approach.

See WASH-BACK METHODS on Page 153

METHAMPHETAMINE (ICE) SMOKING PIPES

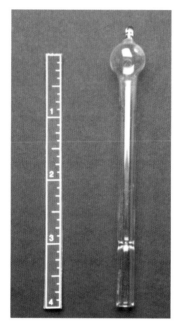

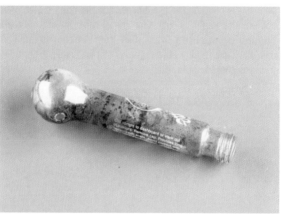

A commercial auto air freshener is emptied and the end of the tube is heated and blown into, creating a bulge at the end. A hole is poked through the bulging end with a hot needle.

METHAMPHETAMINE (ICE) SMOKING PIPES

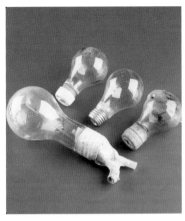

The end of a light bulb is cut off and the insides discarded. A hole is poked in the round end with a hot needle

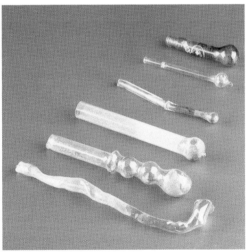

A small piece of the drug is placed inside the round portion of the pipe. The round portion is then heated from beneath, which causes creates vapors. There is a small hole at the top of the round portion of the pipe. The user places a finger over the hole, allowing the vapors to accumulate. The finger is then removed and the vapor is drawn into the lungs. Meth smokers often have a round burn mark on the finger used to block the bowl.

BINDLE

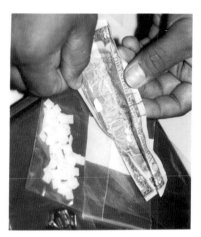

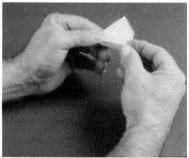

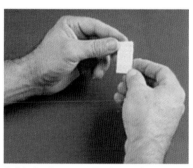

A bindle is a small piece of paper or currency, folded like an envelope to form a pocket, used to hold a personal amount of a drug.

COCAINE SIFTER

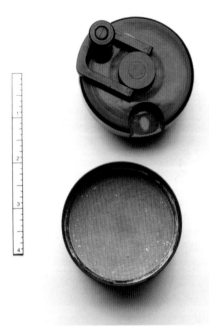

The drug is placed in the top compartment. The lid is screwed on and the handle is turned, forcing the powder through the screen. The result is a powder with a very fine texture for snorting.

SNORTING COCAINE

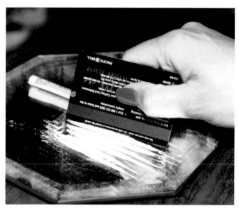

Powdered cocaine is placed on a mirror, piece of glass or other flat, non-porous surface. If not already in fine powder, it may be chopped with a razor blade or credit card. It is then combed into fine lines with the razor or credit card...

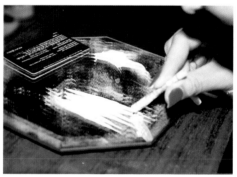

...the lines are then snorted through a tube such as a straw or rolled paper or dollar bill. It may also be snorted with a small spoon.

COPPER SCOURING PADS

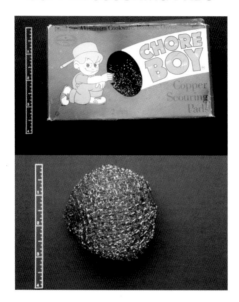

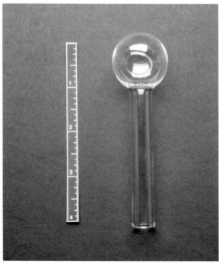

Small, round pieces of these pads are placed in bowls of Freebase Pipes. The "rock" is then placed on top of the pad and lit. The metal fibers of the pad hold the melting **"rock"** and keep it hot. The most popular brand of copper is **"Chore Boy"**. Very fine steel wool or **"Brillo pads"** are also used.

DRUG LAB

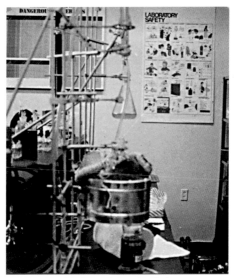

Methamphetamine Lab

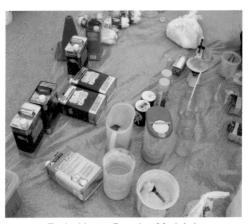

Typical Items Found at Meth Lab

Methamphetamine can be made by a variety of recipes and methods. Simple methods render small quantities and more elaborate productions result in huge quantities. Bottom line, though, the main ingredients are common in households and stores, ephedrine or psuedoephedrine pills, Coleman cooking fuel, lithium batteries (the lithium is removed from the case and is highly flammable), etc.

HEROIN PARAPHERNALIA

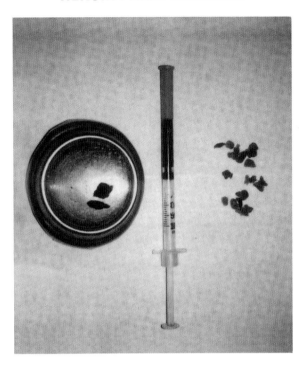

Powdered or Tar Heroin is placed in the "cooker", water is added, and solution is heated. A piece of cotton is added to act as a filter and the solution is drawn up into the needle. The arm is then "tied-off" with a belt, cord, or bandana to bulge the vein. The bulging of the vein is for easy injection and to cause the "rush" after the "tie-off" is released.

The "cooker" is most often made from a spoon or bottom of an aluminum drink can.

This injection process is the same for Cocaine and/or Methamphetamine injections except the drugs are not heated because they are water soluble. They are placed in the cooker and warm water is added.

The "cottons" are kept. When the user does not have drugs, he will use the "cottons" to extract what ever small amount of Heroin is left in them. Cottons are considered drug residue and are not against the law to possess in some states.

NITROUS OXIDE PARAPHERNALIA

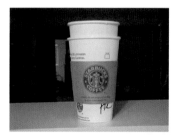 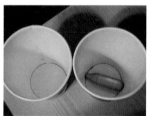

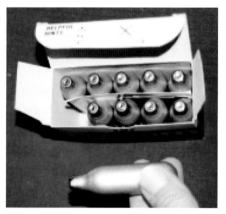

Whippits

Nitrous oxide canisters (smaller than CO2 cylinders) are common in gourmet coffee shops because they propel the whipped cream from homemade whipped cream containers. Nitrous can be abused from the store's whipped cream makers just as it can from commercial cans of whipped cream (holding the can down releases whipped cream, holding it up releases the propellant, nitrous oxide). Employees have been known to slip a canister or two in the bottom of a large cup and then double cup the drink to send nitrous out with a friend

(cont'd next pg.)

NITROUS OXIDE PARAPHERNALIA

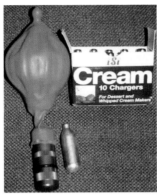

Balloon & Cracker
w/Nitrous Oxide Cartridge

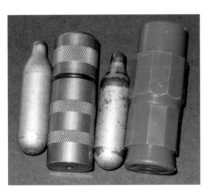
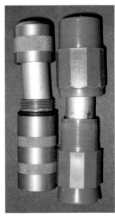

"Crackers" are devices used to puncture the whippets and fill balloons with nitrous oxide to then inhale. Most are aluminum or brass and the manufacturing quality resembles flashlights used by police. But they also come in plastic and can be made from standard PVC fittings (described on the Internet). The balloons are heavy duty, not typical party balloon quality. With the larger tanks of nitrous oxide (from dental offices, dental supply houses or the medium size from high performance vehicle shops), abusers may use the top half of a 2-liter soda bottle as an inhalation mask, attaching it to the tank with a piece of tubing. Inhaling directly from the tanks is dangerous as nitrous oxide gets very cold and can cause damage to lungs, etc. from the intense cold.

RAVE PARAPHERNALIA

MDMA (Ecstasy) enhances all of the senses, making everything pleasurable, including loud noises (users will cling to the speakers for the sound and vibration), touch (may fondle ordinary surfaces and find them fascinating), smell (love the smell of methanol chest rubs to enhance the act of breathing), sights (fascinated by flashing lights, for example), etc.

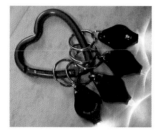
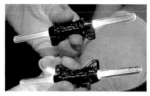

Ravers give each other "light shows" with various spinning or flashing lights. Using the photon lights, visible up to one mile, in their eyes at close proximity may cause damage.

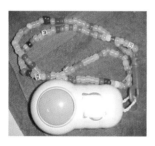
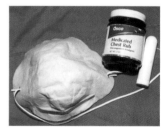

Vibrators, massages, the odor of vapor rub enhances their pleasure.

(cont'd next pg.)

RAVE PARAPHERNALIA

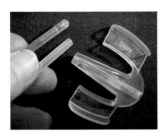
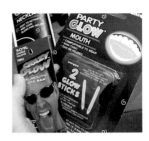

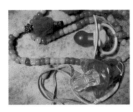
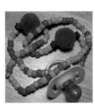

MDMA causes bruxism, teeth grinding; users suck on lollipops, pacifiers, glow sticks, etc., to try to reduce the teeth grinding and jaw locking.

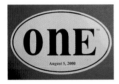
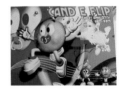

Rave flyers are coded with images or phrases familiar to them and often overlooked by police, teachers and parents. The flyer doesn't say ONE, it says, "On Ecstasy;" Note the lower case "o" and "n" but the capital "E." C and E Flip refers to the flip (practice of mixing MDMA with another drug) of using both LSD and MDMA. "E" or "X" will be highlighted, underlined, capitalized, etc., to accentuate it.

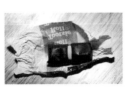

Regular containers may be used to hide their drugs. PEZ containers may harbor MDMA pills or may contain actual PEZ candy laced with liquid LSD. MDMA pills may be found pressed into Tootsie Roll candies to get them past the eyes of teachers, cops and parents. These have also been used to smuggle black tar heroin into jail facilities. MDMA pills have been found intermingled with the candies on candy necklaces.

SCALES

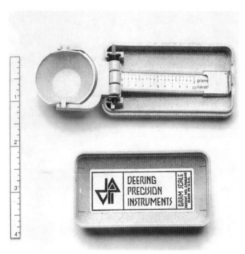

Pocket Drug-Weighing Scale

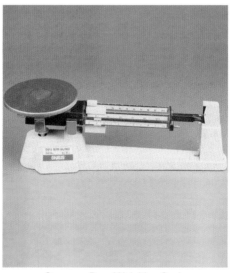

Common Drug Weighing Scale

These scales are often used by dealers who sell in small quantities (such as a gram). The dealers are often called **"Pocket Dealers"**. The scale is assembled and the amount desired is set on the slide arm. The drug is then added to the bowl until the arm is level.

SNORTING SPOON

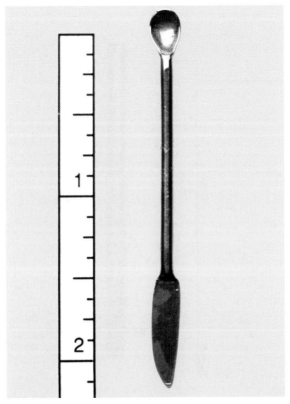

The desired amount of the drug is placed in the bowl of spoon (top in this photo). One nostril is closed while the other nostril is used to snort the drug from the spoon.

SNORTING TUBE

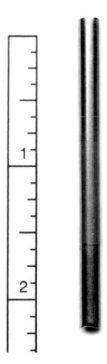

The desired amount of the drug is placed on a smooth surface, such as a piece of glass or a mirror. A razor blade or straight edge, such as a credit card, is used to chop the drug into fine particles. A **"line"** is then made with the substance. The tube is placed into one nostril while the other nostril is closed. The drug is then snorted through the tube into the nose.

Snorting tubes may be made from glass or metal tubing. Often they are made from a tightly rolled twenty dollar bill, which results in the presence of drug residue on the bill.

SNORTING VIALS

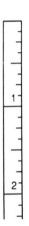
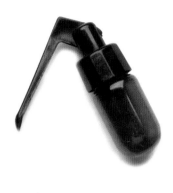

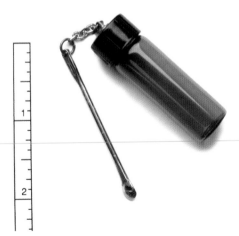

(cont'd next pg.)

SNORTING VIALS

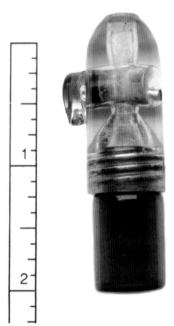

The snorting vial consists of a small vial with a spoon-like device attached to the top. The drug is carried in the vial and a small amount is placed in the "spoon". One nostril is closed and the drug is snorted into the other nostril. In the device above, a small bowl is drilled into the top and the drug is snorted from that bowl.

STASH CANS

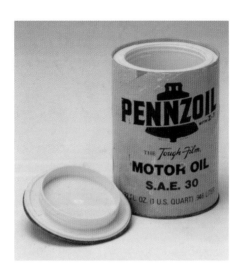

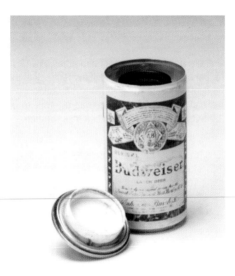

(cont'd next pg.)

STASH CANS

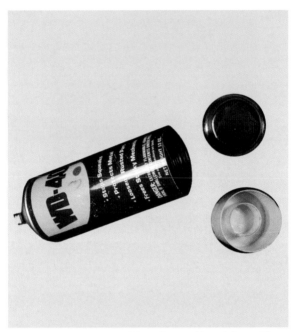

These cans are used to hold small quantities of drugs. Name brand product cans are modified to allow removal of the top or bottom end of the can. Threads may be "reversed" which makes the can appear normal when an attempt to unscrew the end by twisting in a counter-clockwise rotation.

Stash cans may include beer or soft drink cans, aerosol containers, shaving cream cans or any number of other common household products.

WASH-BACK METHODS

As cocaine vapors travel the length of the pipe, some of the vapors dry and adhere to the sides of the pipe. The following processes are popular street methods for retrieving usable cocaine that is trapped inside the pipe.

WET WASH METHOD:

A small amount of "151" rum is put into the mouthpiece of the pipe and the inside is washed out. The rum is then poured on a mirror or a piece of glass and ignited, burning off some of the rum. A piece of copper pad, Brillo pad or steel wool is rubbed on the glass to soak up what is left after burning. The pad is then placed in the pipe, lit, and the vapors drawn into the lungs.

DRY WASH METHOD:

A small amount of "151" rum is put into the mouthpiece of the pipe and the inside is washed out. The rum is then poured on a mirror or a piece of glass and ignited. The rum is burned until it is completely dry. What is left on the glass or mirror is usable cocaine. This residue is scraped off the glass, placed in the pipe and smoked.

The Dry Wash method is the most popular. These Wash-Back methods are primarily used with a freebase cocaine pipe, but may also be used with an "ice" or methamphetamine pipe.

CLOTHING INDICATES DRUG PREFERENCE

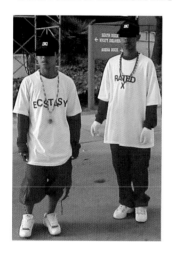 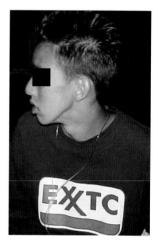

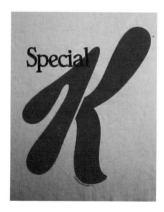

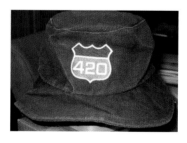

There is an endless stream of clothing and logos indicating drug preference and covers all drugs. Note the Ecstasy, Rated X and EXXTC, all indicating love for the drug MDMA. Special K refers to the animal tranquilizer ketamine. "420" stands for marijuana, April 20 being the universal beginning of the marijuana growing season.

CLOTHES THAT HIDE DRUGS

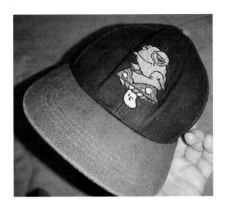

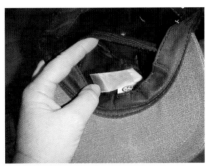

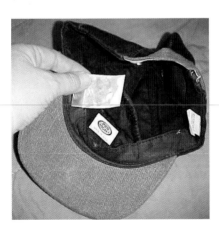

It isn't just in the hat band any more. Hats are made with hidden compartments in the area behind the logo, opening from inside the band with Velcro. Others have entire top sections with Velcro entry on the inside.

(cont'd next pg.)

155

CLOTHES THAT HIDE DRUGS

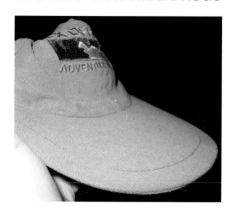

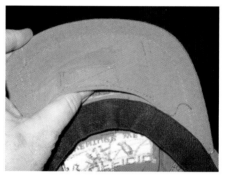

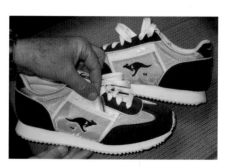

These items are innocent in themselves but it is important to do a thorough search and anticipate unusual hiding spots. Shoes have been found with carved-out areas in the sole, under the insert (commercially made as well as homemade) and in the side zip pockets (styles/brands common for kids and large enough for little more than a key or small quantities of dope. One pair was found at a rave with a zipper completely around the tongue, opening to a large compartment.

CLOTHES THAT HIDE DRUGS

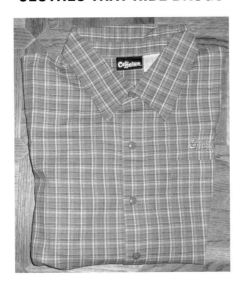

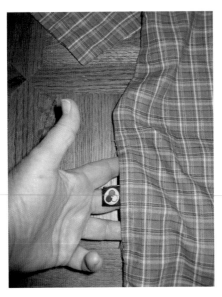

Shirts and pants also come with numerous hidden features. Caffeine brand clothing features the "e" at the end backwards in their logo, similar to the concept of "flipping E," meaning doing the drug Ecstasy with other drugs—poly drug use. Caffeine and Kikwear clothing brands cater to the rave crowd. Velcro pockets may be found in the side seams or hem of shirts and pants. Some pants feature a hidden Velcro compartment on the inner leg seam, for example.

This page intentionally left blank.

NEEDLE INJECTIONS/
PUNCTURE WOUNDS

STERILE INJECTIONS

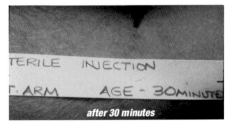

after 30 minutes

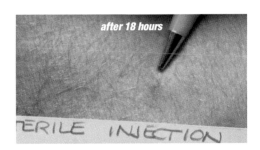

after 18 hours

UNSTERILE INJECTIONS

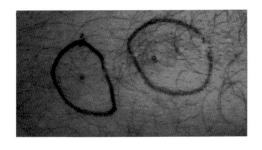

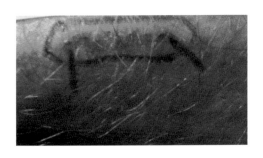

NEEDLE INJECTIONS

Heroin addicts prefer injecting directly into the vein for the most rapid, intense high. Physicians, on the other hand, most commonly inject narcotics under the skin or in muscle. The addict will inject virtually anywhere, either to attempt to hide the marks from view or because the scarring that builds up from chronic use necessitates venturing far and wide to find injection sites. They typically start with the arm and back of the hand but eventually may use ankles, calves, thighs, the groin area, lower portion of the lip, etc. Done properly and with sterile equipment, the injection side will be minor and heal quickly. But, most heroin addicts have marks, scabs, abscesses and scar tissue over their veins from repeated injections under non-sterile, non-hygienic circumstances.

After the "fix" a small pinkish swelling will occur at the injection point. The swelling may appear as a tiny hole and may have fresh blood around it. Within 24 hours an infection may set in from non-sterile conditions. After a day so, the clotting blood and body serums form an orange-pink scab. The first scab would be slightly smaller than the head of a pin, round in shape with raised pink tissue in the center. There may be a bruised area around it if the user is inexperienced or careless. There may be an elongated area if a dull or bent needle was used. If the needle was dirty, there may be a black or blue tinge from the dirt or soot from the needle having been heated with a match. The surrounding tissue may be reddened and could have significant swelling. Two or three days later, the scab will become more orange and swelling reduced. The scab darkens as it ages. After about ten days the scab may flake off. There may be multiple marks of about the same age if the user injects repeatedly throughout the day or misses and has to try again. If the same site is used repeatedly, the scab will be larger and the area more traumatized. Scarring can become significant, forming visible "tracks" of the users historical injection sites. Abscesses may form from the unsanitary conditions and veins can collapse from the ongoing abuse.

Over the years, fear of needles and the growing risk of contracting HIV and other diseases made heroin abuse less attractive to the younger and richer set. But the availability of smokable, black tar heroin caused an increase in heroin abuse in wider circles.

This page intentionally left blank.

APPENDIX

AUTOEROTIC ASPHYXIATION, THE CHOKING GAME & CUTTING

Description:

These are practices gaining attention and perhaps increasing in the United States. The desired result is similar to the practice of inhaling—cutting off oxygen to the brain, for as little as sixty seconds, to produce a brief, euphoric altered state of consciousness that some people find pleasurable.

"Autoerotic Asphyxiation" is the act of masturbating and simultaneously choking oneself or being choked into a state of unconsciousness, enhancing sensation. "Erotic Asphyxiation" refers to couples choking each other during sexual acts for enhancement. This is a dangerous practice as the asphyxiation may go too far, resulting in injury or death.

"The Choking Game" has become increasingly popular among youth and is somewhat similar to inhalant abuse as it provides a brief euphoric experience. It's the younger version of sexual practice noted above. They call it things like, "fainting each other" or "dreaming." It produces a brief high and can cause brain damage or death. Indicators are unusual marks around the neck; ties, ropes or belts in unusual configurations; complaints of headaches; blood shot eyes.

"Cutting" or self-mutilation or other forms of self-harm is the act of seeking an altered mood state by inflicting harm serious enough to cause tissue damage to one's own body. It is a non-verbal means of dealing with overwhelming feelings or situations.

DRUG-FACILITATED SEXUAL ASSAULTS

Drug-Facilitated Sexual Assault **(DFSA)** is an offender's use of "anesthesia-type" drugs or hallucinogens, whether given stealthily or not, to render a subject physically helpless or otherwise incapacitated and thus incapable of giving or withholding consent. Voluntary intoxication does NOT equal consent to have sex, though it does represent risky behavior and leave the person more vulnerable to assault. The various drugs used in DFSA have a variety of effects with the most prevalent being intoxication, amnesia, sleepiness or unconsciousness, and general inability to control their environment. The victim may be unconscious during all or part of act, and may have amnesia even when conscious and appearing to function and "participate" at some stages.

More than 40 different drugs have been used to facilitate sexual assault (and may also be used in robbery). Predatory drugs include these types of drugs:

- Alcohol
- GHB or its "analogs" GBL, BD and others
- Benzodiazepines, such as flunitrazepam (roofies, Rohypnol), Ativan, Xanax, etc.
- Other sedative-hypnotics, such as ketamine, PCP
- Sleeping pills, such as Ambien
- Muscle relaxants, such as Soma, Flexeril
- Antihistamines, such as diphenhydramine (as in Benadryl)
- Animal tranquilizers, such telazol
- Motion sickness/nausea prevention pills, such as scopalomine
- Narcotic analgesics
- MDMA & other hallucinogens

Urine is the sample of choice in DFSA cases and should be obtained as soon as possible, as some of these drugs dissipate from the body rapidly. GHB, for example, is in the blood for only four hours and in the urine for only 12.

Absence of a drug in toxicology results alone does not mean that a drug rape has not occurred. Consider the timing of the event—the time from the suspected drink or food and the time when the sample was finally obtained. A negative toxicology result may merely reflect that the sample was taken after the drug dissipated. The victim's statements, observations by witnesses, etc., may help to establish that a drug, and which drug type, was likely used. Some state laws do not require a positive test result proving a specific drug but may be prosecuted based on effects, observed symptoms, etc. Screening tests may NOT detect all drugs. Confirmation testing should be done when circumstances indicate a possible DFSA and the drug screen is negative.

DRUG STATISTICS

DEA Drug Seizures					
Calender Year	Cocaine kgs	Heroin kgs	Marijuana kgs	Meth kgs	Hallucinogen dosage units
2008	49,823.3	598.6	660,969.2	1540.4	9,199,693
2007	96,713	625	356,472	1,086	5,636,305
2006	69,826	805	322,438	1,711	4,606,277
2005	118,270	639	282,139	2,148.6	8,861,503
2004	117,847	672	265,810	1,653.5	2,483,702
2003	73,718	789	254,241	1,676.9	2,879,543
2002	63,640	710	238,646	1,352.8	11,661,811
2001	59,428	753	271,918	1,634.1	13,769,190
2000	58,674	546	331,499	1,771.4	29,307,721
1999	36,165	351	338,287	1,488.8	1,736,118
1998	34,448	371	262,244	1,202.7	1,075,457
1997	28,670	399	215,424	1,143.2	1,100,912
1996	44,735	320	192,132	751.0	1,720,153
1995	45,327	877	219,830	875.1	2,774,376
1994	74,850	491	157,203	767.6	1,367,679
1993	55,655	616	143,056	559.8	2,710,063
1992	69,324	722	201,513	352.7	1,305,208
1991	67,002	1,174	98,620	289.6	1,297,395
1990	60,932	541	133,672	274.5	2,826,966
1989	73,562	758	286,372	896.0	13,125,010
1988	60,951	728	347,306	693.8	16,706,442
1987	49,683	515	629,860	198.6	6,559,317
1986	29,389	421	491,831	234.5	4,146,329

Source: DEA (STRIDE)

DRUG STATISTICS

DEA Arrests (Domestic)	
Calendar Year	**Number of Arrests**
2008	26,425
2007	29,097
2006	29,993
2005	28,828
2004	29,952
2003	28,549
2002	30,270
2001	34,471
2000	39,743
1999	41,293
1998	38,468
1997	34,068
1996	29,269
1995	25,279
1994	23,135
1993	21,637
1992	24,541
1991	23,659

Source: DEA (SMARTS)
Defendant Statistical System (DSS)

DRUG STATISTICS

Total of All Meth Clandestine Laboratory Incidents
Including Labs, Dumpsites, Chem/Glass/Equipment
Calendar Year 2008

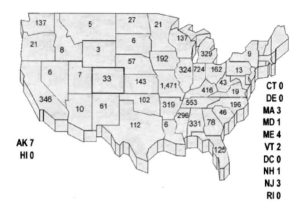

Source: National Clandestine Laboratory Database
Total: 6783
Dates: 01/01/2008 - 12/31/2008

Drug Enforcement Administration Heroin Signature Program

The DEA operates the Heroin Signature Program (HSP), using scientific profiling to identify the origin of heroin seized and purchased in the United States. DEA chemists can determine which of the world's four major heroin producing regions was the source of the drug. These regions are: South America, Mexico, Southeast Asia and Southwest Asia. HSP data is used in conjunction with investigative intelligence and with production and seizure data to develop an overall assessment of heroin trafficking to and within the United States. More information is available at the DEA website: **www.dea.gov.**

EARLY WARNING SIGNS
Early Warning Signs of Adolescent Drug Abuse

There are numerous early warning signs of adolescent drug abuse. In order to detect the early warning signs, keep an open line of communication and be aware, observant, and open-minded. Drug abuse infiltrates all social, economic, and cultural structures. The current national average of the onset of drug and alcohol use is under 13 years of age.

EARLY WARNING SIGNS:

1. A distinctive change in attitude, usually a negative change.
2. Decline in school work and grades.
3. Poor school attendance, frequent Monday and Friday absences.
4. Distinctive change in friends.
5. Distinctive change in clothing.
6. Distinctive change in taste of music and movies.
7. Disciplinary problems a home and school.
8. Isolation from friends.
9. Mood swings.
10. Outbursts of violence (physical and/or verbal).
11. Discovery of drugs, drug paraphernalia, or drug publications.
12. Distinctive change in appearance. (Examples: tattoos, ear rings, nose rings, etc.)
13. Noticeable decrease in motivation and enthusiasm.
14. Abandonment of areas of interest or hobbies.
15. Stealing (inside and outside the home).
16. Marked increase of physical illness.

GATEWAY DRUGS

Gateway drugs are most commonly used by adolescents. These drugs are:

- Alcohol
- Tobacco (including smokeless)
- Inhalants

Adolescence is the life stage between childhood and adulthood. The onset of gateway drug use was considered to be around age 12 yrs., but is often younger. Adolescents use the so-called gateway drugs due to the fact they are readily available and inexpensive. These chemicals can cause inhibition of growth and abnormal emotional development. They reason they are called gateway drugs is that they can lead the adolescent down the path toward other illicit drug abuse.

More recently MDMA (Ecstasy) has become a major gateway drug and rave parties are often a "gateway event" for the young. The first drug they are exposed to—whatever drug that is—may be the gateway, opening the door to other drug exposure and usage. Parents may serve as the gateway, especially with alcohol, tobacco and today with methamphetamine.

DRUG EVALUATION & TESTING

PUPIL/LIGHT ACCOMMODATION TEST

The purpose of this series of tests is to examine the reaction, or lack of reaction, to the presence and absence of light. Use a pen light and a Pupilometer. (Average pupil size is 3.0 to 6.5 millimeters.)

AVAILABLE LIGHT

Using whatever light is available at the time of the test, use a Pupilometer to check the size of both pupils. Always check the left pupil first (to keep the test standardized and systematic) and note the size of each pupil separately. To do this, place the Pupilometer along the temple side of the eye. Locate the circle that best matches the size of the pupil and note that size. (Do not cover any portion of the eye with the Pupilometer during this test.)

CLOSE TO TOTAL DARKNESS

Expose the subject's eyes to a minimum of 90 seconds of uninterrupted, total darkness. Next, place the pad of the index finger over the lens of the pen light. (This will result in a red light.) Place the Pupilometer on the temple side of the eye and shine the red light into the eye. Measure the size of the pupil, doing the left eye first (to keep the test standardized and systematic), then note the size of each pupil separately.

INDIRECT LIGHT

Using the white light of the pen light, illuminate the temple about 6 inches away from the side of the head. Bring inner beam of light forward until it shines across the front of eyeball, creating a shadow or silhouette on the side of the nose halfway between the corner of the eye and the bridge of the nose. Place Pupilometer beside the left eye first (to standardize test) and measure the size of the pupil of each eye separately. (Do not shade the light with the Pupilometer.)

DIRECT LIGHT

Shine the inner beam of the pen light directly into the eye. Position the beam of light between the eyebrows and the top of the cheekbone. Hold the light in this position for one minute. Measure the size of the pupil of the left eye first (to standardize test) with the Pupilometer. Note the measurement of each pupil separately.

(cont'd next pg.)

HORIZONTAL NYSTAGMUS TEST

SMOOTH PURSUIT

While the subject is looking straight ahead, place a stimulus (index finger) 15 inches in front of the tip of the nose and even with the eyebrows. Move the stimulus (index finger) to the subject's left about 45 degrees watching for an involuntary jerking of the eyes. Proceed to move the stimulus (index finger) to the right eye and repeat procedure. Do this twice with each eye. When moving the stimulus (index finger) to the left, check the left eye. When moving the stimulus (index finger) to the right, check the right eye. Move the stimulus (index finger) straight across in front of the subject's face.

MAXIMUM DEVIATION

Administer this test in the exact same manner as the Smooth Pursuit Test except at the 45 degrees, hold the stimulus (index finger) still for 5 seconds. Look for involuntary jerking of the eye.

Additional Comments:

Some people have nystagmus naturally.

Vertical Nystagmus Test

With the subject looking straight ahead, place the stimulus (index finger) 15 inches out from the tip of the nose. Move stimulus (index finger) upward level with the top of the head and down to the tip of the nose. Do this test at least twice looking at each eye once. Record your results.

NOTE: Vertical Nystagmus is when the eyeballs jerk vertically (up and down).

Non-Convergence Test

When the subject is looking straight ahead, place the stimulus (index finger) 15 inches in front of the tip of the nose. First move the stimulus in front of the face counter clockwise. The circles should not be larger than the subject's face.

When you are sure the subject is following the stimulus with his eyes, bring the stimulus (index finger) to the nose and touch the bridge of the nose. Tell the subject to watch the stimulus (index finger) on the bridge of the nose for at least 5 seconds. Look for either or both eyes drifting outward, not being able to focus inward on the nose.

Additional Comments:

Non-convergence can be natural in some individuals.

(cont'd next pg.)

STANDARD FIELD SOBRIETY TESTS

The following is an explanation of the four standardized field sobriety tests. Please keep in mind:

1. These tests should be used for **ALL** drug influence situations, not just for alcohol intoxication.

2. Give clear instructions to the subject and be sure they understand what is required of them before they begin each test.

3. Conduct each test on a flat surface that is well-lighted and void of any obstructions.

4. Discontinue any test if the subject is in any danger of injury.

5. Take complete notes as you administer each test.

6. These tests should be given in the same order and instructed in the same way each time to standardize the tests.

RHOMBERG 30 SECOND ESTIMATION OF TIME

During the explanation and demonstration of this test, have the subject stand upright with heels and toes together and their hands at their sides. This is the "Rhomberg Position."

TEST: In the "Rhomberg Position," have the subject tilt his head back and close his eyes. When you say begin, have the subject estimate 30 seconds. (This should be done silently.) When the subject believes the 30 seconds are finished, he should open his eyes and bring his head forward. This indicates the end of the test. If the subject has not completed the test in 90 seconds, discontinue the test.

Additional Comments:

1. Drugs that speed up the body will cause a short estimation of time (cocaine, amphetamines, etc.), and the drugs that slow the system down will cause a long estimation of time (depressants, narcotics, alcohol, etc.).

2. Be aware of the actual time during the test. Note body movements such as swaying, body tremors, muscle rigidity, etc.

3. Make sure the subject performs the test as instructed.

(cont'd next pg.)

WALK-AND-TURN

During the explanation and demonstration, have the subject place his right foot on the line he will be walking on. Then have him place the toes of his left foot against the heel of his right foot. Standing flat on the ground with both feet pointing in the same direction, stand up straight with both arms at his side.

TEST: After assuming the above position, instruct the subject to walk nine steps up the line, turn around and walk nine steps back. (Each step should be heel to toe.) The subject will look down at his feet and count each step out loud. At the end of the first nine steps, the subject will turn. (The turn will be a three-point pivot), keeping the front foot in its place and using the balls of this foot to pivot.) With the back foot, push three times around to face the opposite direction. Walk back nine steps in the same manner. If at any time the subject falls off the line, he is to regain his balance and continue to walk and count off his steps where he left off. Discontinue test if subject is in danger of injury.

Additional Comments:

1. Note any difficulties balancing.

2. Note if the subject uses his arms or any other object for balance.

3. Be sure he touches heel to toe as instructed.

4. Make sure the turn is done as instructed.

5. The counting of steps should be loud enough to be heard.

6. Make sure the subject performs the test as instructed.

ONE-LEG-STAND

During the explanation and demonstration, have the subject stand in the "Rhomberg Position." (Stand upright with heels and toes together, and hands at the side.)

TEST: From the "Rhomberg Position," instruct the subject to first balance on his left leg by raising his right leg until his right foot is six inches off the ground. Have the subject point his toes down on the right foot, and while looking at his right foot, count to 30 out loud. (Have the subject count one thousand one, one thousand two, one thousand three, etc.) If at any time the subject loses his balance, he is to regain balance and continue counting where he left off. Discontinue test if subject is in danger of injury.

Additional Comments:

1. Note if subject uses arms or any other object for balance.

2. Note any difficulties in balancing.

3. The subject must count correctly.

4. Make sure the subject performs the test as instructed.

(cont'd next pg.)

FINGER-TO-NOSE

During the explanation and demonstration, the subject should stand in the "Rhomberg Position." (Stand upright with heels and toes together, and hands at the side.) Have the subject make a fist with both hands and extend his index finger on each hand, then place his arms at his sides.

TEST: From the above position, instruct the subject to tilt his head back and close his eyes. When instructed, the subject is to touch the tip of his index finger to the tip of his nose. After touching his nose, the subject will bring his hand down to the starting position without being told. The sequence of instruction is left, right, left, right, right, left.

Additional Comments:

1. Note any body movements, such as swaying, body tremors, muscle rigidity, etc.

2. Observe where the index finger touches the face.

3. Make sure the subject performs the test as instructed.

DRUG TESTING

BODY FLUIDS REQUIRED FOR TESTING

Choice of body fluid will depend on a variety of considerations, including the drug that is suspected and the timing of when the sample is being taken. With alcohol, blood or breath is preferred. If, however, other drugs are involved, urine may be preferred. If the suspect is clearly under the influence, blood may be an appropriate choice, as in drunk/drugged driving cases where the subject is still under the influence at the time the sample is taken. With possible drug-facilitated sexual assault cases, urine is always the preferred sample. If collection is being made within a few hours of the suspected drugging, blood may be worthwhile, and could be taken in addition to a urine sample.

Blood and urine have both advantages and disadvantages. The presence of drugs in blood is more closely related to impairment, but may be more difficult to obtain (requiring specially trained personnel) and is often more expensive to analyze. Urine is easier to obtain and the concentration of drugs and metabolites in urine is often easier to detect. Drugs remain in urine longer than in blood. Taking urine specimens may allow the subject a greater opportunity to tamper with the sample contents (adding someone else's urine, diluting the sample, etc,).

UNDERSTANDING TOXICOLOGY RESULTS

Toxicology results can be confusing as they may be reported in a variety of concentration units. They may be reported as nanograms per milliliter (ng/mL). Other labs use micrograms per milliliter (μg/mL). There is a 1,000-time difference between nanograms and micrograms, making comparison and understand very confusing.

UNITS OF CONCENTRATION CONVERSION

1 mg/L	=	1 μg/mL
1 mg/mL	=	1000 ug/mL
1 μg/mL	=	1000 ng/mL
1 mg/dL	=	10 μg/mL
100 μg/dL	=	1 μg/mL

DETECTION LIMITS

Note: Times relate to length of time drugs can be detected in urine, except where blood limitations are specifically noted. Times are estimates and specific drugs within categories may vary.

Cocaine .... 2-3 days
Metabolite*

Cannabis
Single use .... 3 days
Moderate use (4 times/week) .... 5 days
Heavy use (daily) .... 10 days
Chronic heavy use........... 21-27 days

Gamma Hydroxybutyrate (GHB & Analogs GBL & BD)
Urine...................... 12 hours
Blood .... 3-5 hours

Opiates...................... 48 hours
(including heroin, morphine, codeine)

PCP (Phencyclidine) ... 48 hours to 8 days

Amphetamines .... 48 hours
(including methamphetamines)
Benzodiazepines** .... 3 days, approx
(including diazepam/Valium, clonazepam/Klonopins, therapeutic dose)

Barbiturates
Short acting (secobarbital) .... 24 hours
Intermediate acting .... 48-72 hours
Long acting (phenobarbital) .. 7 days or more
Phenobarbital .... 24 hours (blood)

Propoxyphene (Darvon)
Unchanged .... 6 hours
Metabolite* .... 6-48 hours

(cont'd next pg.)

DETECTION LIMITS

*A metabolite is the substance(s) produced by the body metabolizing (breaking down) a drug. Metabolites may by psychoactive or inactive, but are detectable in blood and urine and are often the basis for drug tests. For example, cocaine produces the metabolite benzoylecogonine; when cocaethylene (aka: ethylcocaine) is detected, that indicates combined use of alcohol and cocaine. Presence of the parent drug, cocaine, indicates recent use. Some drugs are detected only as the drug itself, with no metabolites, such as PCP.

**There is a wide range of benzodiazepine drugs available and some may not be readily detectable in a "drug screen" (i.e. immunoassay) in either blood or urine, such as lorazepam (Ativan), alprazolam (Xanax) and triazolam (Halcion). Other testing procedures should be used before ruling out the presence of benzos.

WEIGHTS & MEASURES

DRY MEASURES

1 Microgram (mcg.)	=	1/1000 of a Milligram (mg.)
1000 Micrograms (mcg.)	=	1 Milligram (mg.)
1000 Grams	=	1 Kilogram (kilo.)
1 Kilogram (kilo.)	=	2.2 Pounds (lbs.)
1 Gram (g.)	=	15.43 Grains (gr.)
28.35 Grams (g.)	=	1 Ounce (oz.)
453.6 Grams (g.)	=	1 Pound (lb.)
1 Grain (gr.)	=	65 Milligrams (mg.)
1 Grain (gr.)	=	.065 Grams (g.)
1 Ounce (oz.)	=	437.5 Grains (gr.)
1 Ounce (oz.)	=	28.3 Grams (g.)
1 Ounce (oz.)	=	28,350 Milligrams (mg.)
1 Ounce (oz.)	=	6 Tablespoons (tbls.) approx.
1 Pound (lbs.)	=	7,000 Grains
1 Pound (lbs.)	=	16 Ounces
1 Pound (lbs.)	=	453 Grams (g.)
1 Ton	=	2,000 Pounds (lbs.)

LIQUID MEASURES

1 L (Liter)	=	approximately one quart
1000ml (milliliters)	=	1 Liter

Additional Comments:

For comparison purposes and for training, one gram equals one packet of sugar substitute, such as Sweet N Low.

179

DRUG ABUSE IN THE WORKPLACE

STATISTICS:

1. An estimated 70% of all individuals abusing drugs are employed.

2. The abuse of alcohol and other drugs is costing American business owners over one hundred billion dollars ($100,000,000, 000) annually due to insurance rate increases, workman's compensation, etc.

3. Drug use shows up at all levels in the workplace, from professionals to unskilled workers.

4. An estimated 20% of the workplace population is using alcohol or other drugs at the work-site.

5. Almost 60% of the world's production of illegal drugs are consumed in the United States while only 5% of the world's population is located in the United States.

ABUSERS IN THE WORKPLACE:

1. Are less productive.

2. Miss several days of work.

3. Are more likely to injure themselves or someone else.

4. File more worker's compensation claims.

5. Are more likely to steal from employer and/or co-workers.

6. A cause of low morale among co-workers.

7. Cause an increase in co-worker's work load.

8. Cause insurance rates to increase.

RECOGNIZING ABUSERS IN THE WORKPLACE:

1. Accidents on the job.

2. Frequent absences and/or late to work.

3. Frequent mistakes that require additional work to correct.

4. Uncharacteristic behavior (moodiness, giddiness, violent threats, etc.).

5. Obsessed with drugs and alcohol and trying to get others to participate.

FIGHTING DRUG ABUSE IN THE WORKPLACE

The best way to fight drug abuse in the workplace is through a five part program.

1. A written substance abuse policy.

2. An employee education & awareness program.

3. Supervisor training program.

4. An employee assistance program.

5. Drug testing when appropriate.

WORKPLACE DRUG ABUSE RESOURCES

California Narcotic Officers' Association
(877) 775-6272
www.cnoa.org

American Council for Drug Education
(800) 488-DRUG (3784)
(301) 394-0600

Drug-Free Workplace Helpline
(800) WORKPLACE 9am to 8 pm EST
www.health.org/workpl.htm

National Clearinghouse for
Alcohol & Drug Information
(800) 729-6686

National Institute on Drug Abuse
Treatment (NIDA) Hotline
(800) 662-HELP (4357)

The Resource Center for Alcohol
and Drug Problems
(800) 879-2772

SAMHSA Treatment Facilities Locator
http://dasis3.samhsa.gov/

Resources for Drug Prevention

www.projectghb.org

www.taylorhooton.org

www.couragetospeak.org

www.notMYkid.org

www.dammad.org

www.painfullyobvious.com

www.teens.drugabuse.gov

www.theantidrug.com

www.drugfree.org

www.justthinktwice.com

This page intentionally left blank.

DEFINITIONS

ANABOLIC STEROID   Medically used to some extent but also personally abused to promote muscle growth and tissue development. Typically abused by athletes but increased use has been seen among teens to overcome harassment for being small, skinny and by young females to be more firm and lean. Users run the risk of increased cancer, acne and other negative side effects. Many counterfeit products are also being distributed.

ANALGESIC   Drugs that relieve pain, such as codeine, zolpidem, oxycodone, etc.

ANALOG   Chemical cousin of another drug, with similar properties and related chemical structure (definition for legal purposes varies from state to state). This is the basis for "designer drug" issues, where a chemist may alter the structure of an illegal substance, seeking a drug of similar properties for abuse purposes but not yet illegal. But, when and where analog laws apply (and depending on the precise wording), the new substance may be automatically covered and made illegal for human consumption.

ATAXIA   Loss of muscle coordination.

CNS   Central Nervous System.

HYPERTHERMIA   Over-heating of the body due to certain drug effects or disease. Defined as body temperature over 104 degrees. Drugs associated with this include MDMA, LSD, amphetamines, cocaine, PCP, etc.

HYPOTHERMIA   Decreased body temperature due to exposure to cold, certain drug effects. Defined as body temperature below 90 degrees. Drugs associated with this include barbiturates, ethanol, GHB, sedative-hypnotics, opiates, etc.

SINSEMILLA   Seedless marijuana.

SYNESTHESIA   The effect of drugs such as LSD in which the user's sensory system is crossed, resulting in the "seeing" sounds, "hearing" colors, etc.

TACHYCARDIA   Excessive heart rate (pulse greater than 100).

STREET SLANG

Varies greatly from city to city, state to state, culture to culture, etc. We have attempted to gather the most commonly used language.

2-CI   Emerging street drug 2,5-dimethoxy-4-iodophenethy- lamine (See TRYPTAMINE)

2-CB   Street drug 4-bromo-2,5-dimethoxyphenethylamine (See NEXUS, BROMO)

2C-T-7   Street drug 2,5-dimethoxy-4-(n)-propylthiophenethyl- amine known as Tripstasy, Lucky 7, 7-Up (See LUCKY 7)

8-TRACK   Street gang term meaning 2.5 grams of Cocaine

ABE   Five dollars worth of a drug

ABSINTHE   Typically green liquor of grain alcohol and wormwood (artemesia absinthium), with a high alcohol content plus the chemical thujone

ACAPULCO GOLD   A particularly potent form of Marijuana grown in the Acapulco area (See GOLD and GOLD LEAF)

ACCESSORIES   Drug paraphernalia

ACE   1) A Marijuana cigarette (See JOINT) 2) PCP

ACETONE   A chemical that is mainstay of many illicit drug preparations, making it a regulated chemical; can also be abused as an inhalant

ACID   LSD (Lysergic Acid Diethylamide)

ACID CUBE   A sugar cube containing LSD

ACID FREAK   A heavy regular user of LSD

ACID HEAD   LSD user

ACK-ACK   Method by which Heroin/Cocaine is smoked on the tip of a burning cigarette

ACTION   To use or sell drugs

AD   A drug addict

ADAM   Slang for the drug MDMA (3,4-Methylenedioxy-N-Methylamphetamine)

ADAM & EVE IN THE GARDEN OF EDEN   Polydrug abuse, called a flip, taking MDMA with the drugs MDEA and MBDB, all at the same time (See FLIP)

AFGHANI   Drugs from Afghanistan Usually Marijuana

AMF   Slang for the drug Alpha-Methylfentanyl

AMPED   High on amphetamines

AMBIEN   Sleeping pill containing Zolpidem that can be abused or used for drugging for rape or robbery

AMT/a-MT   Alpha-methyl-tryptamine is another drug being seen in pill or powder form, typically in same clientele as MDMA; also called Spirals, Amtrak or Amthrax (See TRYPTAMINE)

AMYL NITRATE   A prescription drug for coronary artery disease that is also abused by inhaling the fumes, giving a brief but intense rush (See POPPERS, BUTYL NITRATE)

ANABOLIC STEROID   Medically used to some extent but also personally abused to promote muscle growth and tissue development; typically abused by athletes but increased use has been seen among teens to overcome harassment for being small, skinny and by young females to be more firm and lean; users run the risk of increased cancer, acne and other negative side effects; many counterfeit products are also being distributed

ANALGESIC   Drugs that relieve pain, such as codeine, zolpidem, oxycodone, etc.

ANALOG   Chemical cousin of another drug, with similar properties and related chemical structure (definition for legal purposes varies from state to state); this is the basis for "designer drug" issues, where a chemist may alter the structure of an illegal substance, seeking a drug of similar properties for abuse purposes but not yet illegal; when and where analog laws apply (and depending on the precise wording), the new substance may be automatically covered and made illegal for human consumption

ANGEL DUST   **1)** Phencyclidine (PCP) **2)** PCP sprinkled on Marijuana in powdered form and smoked

ANGEL'S TRUMPET   The Datura plant, a hallucinogen, is also called Angel's Trumpet or Devil Weed or Jimson Weed (See DATURA)

ANIMAL TRANK   PCP

ARNOLD   Street term for anabolic steroid

ARTILLERY   Drug paraphernalia for injecting

ASTRO TURF   Marijuana

ATROPINE   From datura and belladonna plants, atropine has legitimate medical uses but abuse can produce hallucinations, severe toxic effects and even death

AUTHOR   A doctor or anyone who writes illegal prescriptions

BABYSITTER   An individual knowledgeable about the effects of hallucinogens, particularly in the case of LSD The babysitter provides reassurance and reality for the novice user (See CO-PILOT)

BACK-UP   A procedure permitting blood back into the syringe to ensure that the needle is in a vein (a frequent precaution taken by veteran heroin addicts)

BAD TRIP   An unpleasant, frightening or even terrifying experience occurring after the ingestion of a hallucinogenic drug or after ingestion of other drugs with hallucinogenic properties

BAG   A small container of a drug, usually just enough for personal use

BALL   Mexican Black Tar Heroin

BALLOON   A toy balloon used for packaging Mexican Powdered Heroin. The balloon is used to enable the possessor to swallow it if approached by the authorities. It is later retrieved after defecation

BANG   Injecting

BARBS   Barbiturates

BARREL   **1)** A quantity of 100,000 pills **2)** A particular shape of LSD tablet

BASA   Spanish word for base

BASE   Freebased Cocaine

BASEBALL   Cocaine Freebase

BASING   The process of converting powdered Cocaine (Hydrochloride) into a purified solid for smoking

BASUCO/BASA   Raw Coca Paste directly from the Coca Plant. It is a dark paste that is smoked, usually by South American peasants

BATU   Hawaiian term for the large smokable crystals of Methamphetamine

BAYONET   Hypodermic syringe

BC   Bud Marijuana from British Columbia

BEANS   1)Dexedrine 2) more currently and commonly used to refer to MDMA pills, especially in Florida

BEAUTIFUL   A drug of good quality, producing an exceptionally intense euphoria

BEHIND STUFF   Using heroin, as in "I'm behind stuff"

BELLY HABIT   Addiction where withdrawals cause severe stomach cramps

BELT   1) High or Euphoria produced by a drug high 2) To quickly consume alcohol 3) A large mouthful of alcohol.

BENNIES   The prescription drug Benzedrine, however, it is no longer manufactured (See BENZ and DRIVERS)

BENT   To be high on any drug

BENZ   The prescription drug Benzedrine, however, it is no longer manufactured (See BENNIES and DRIVERS)

BENZODIAZEPINE (aka: BENZO)   A group of depressant drugs typically for sleep or anxiety disorders, such as Valium, Xanax, Ativan (See DEPRESSANTS)

BERNICE   Cocaine

BETEL NUT   From the areca palm tree, betel nut is commonly used in some Asian cultures and produces a mild stimulant effect

BHANG   Marijuana

BIG CHIEF   Peyote

BIG C   Cocaine

BIG D   LSD

BIG H   Heroin

BIG MAN   Upper level drug dealer

BINDLE   Paper used to hold a personal amount of a powdered drug Folded like an envelope

BINGE   A sustained period of uninterrupted alcohol uses, sometimes refers to the same practice with other drugs

BINKY or BINKIE   Pacifiers used by abusers of the drug MDMA (Ecstasy) to reduce the bruxism (teeth grinding) that it often causes

BLACK & WHITES   Biphetamine that comes in a black & white capsule (See BLACK BEAUTIES)

BLACK BEAUTIES   Biphetamine that comes in a black and white capsule (See BLACK & WHITES)

BLACK JACK   Tincture of Opium cooked to a concentrated form and injected

BLACK TAR HEROIN   A form of Mexican Heroin

BLANK   An inert substance mixed with a drug to produce more of the substance for sales

BLASTED   An intense drug high

BLAZING   Smoking marijuana

BLOND   Gold or yellow colored solid Hashish from the Middle East (Lebanese Blond)

BLOTTER ACID   Small squares of heavy stock paper, perforated for tearing, with a drop of LSD on each. Ingested orally. Sometimes there are pictures stamped on each one.

BLOW   1) Slang for Cocaine **2)** Inhalation of smoke

BLOW A STICK (OR JOINT)   Smoking a marijuana joint

BLOW THE VEIN   Injecting a vein with too much of the substance usually causing the vein to collapse

BLOW YOUR MIND   To get high on a hallucinogenic

BLOWING UP (or BLOWIN' UP)   Getting high on MDMA (Ecstasy)

BLUE CHEER   A combination of LSD, Methamphetamine, and Strychnine

BLUE DEVILS   Prescription drug Amytal Sodium in a blue capsule

BLUE HEAVEN   LSD

BLUELIGHTER   Refers to someone who participates in the on-line message board called bluelight, a common discussion ground for ravers and drug abusers (www.bluelight.nu)

BLUE MYSTIC   Street drug 2C-T-7, also called Triptasy or 7-Up (See TRYPTAMINE)

BLUE NITRO   Common GBL product (GHB analog) disguised as a dietary supplement

BLUES   Amytal Sodium capsule

BLUE STAR   A type of Morning Glory plant. The seeds can cause hallucinations similar to that of LSD

BLUE VELVET   Tincture of Opium added to powdered Tripelennamine, made into a solution and injected for a very intense high

BLUNT   Hollowed out cigar filled with marijuana

BO   Street gang term for Marijuana

BOAT   1,000 MDMA pills; also called a bucket in some regions

BODY CARRIER   Drug smuggler who carries the contraband in their clothes or on their body

BODY PACKER   Drug smuggler who swallows the contraband which is usually wrapped in balloons or condoms. Later it is retrieved after defecation (see MULE)

BOGART   Not sharing any drug

BOMBED   Excessive drug intoxication

BOLIVIAN **1)** Cocaine of the purest form **2)** Country of origin

BOLSA Spanish word for bag. Usually refers to Heroin

BOLT Amyl Nitrite

BONG Marijuana smoking pipe that is usually glass with a cooling chamber that is filled with water or wine

BOWL **1)** Marijuana pipe **2)** A degree measurement of Marijuana

BOTTLE 100 pills

BOY Heroin

BOWL PARTY See PHARMING, TRAIL MIX

BRICK A quantity of Marijuana compressed into the shape of a brick that usually weighs a kilogram (2.2 lbs.)

BRING DOWN **1)** To precipitate a "crash" from the excessive agitation produced by stimulants, via the ingestion of a CNS depressant **2)** To help reduce highly adverse effects produced in some h hallucinogen users via talk, reassurance, and sometimes minor tranquilizers

BRING IT UP To bulge a vein prior to injection

BRODY, TO THROW A To feign illness or withdraw in an attempt to obtain a narcotic prescription from a sympathetic physician

BROTHER Heroin

BROWN STUFF Mexican Brown Powdered Heroin

BROWNIES Regular fudge brownies mixed with Marijuana

BRUXISM Teeth grinding and jaw locking commonly caused by drugs such as MDMA and methamphetamine

BUBBLES 4-methylmethcathinone (See MEPHEDRONE)

BUCKET 1,000 MDMA pills in some regions; more commonly called a boat (See BOAT)

BUD The blossom at the top of the Marijuana plant that contains the highest level of THC which is the active component of the plant

BUDDHA STICK Potent Asian Marijuana which is wrapped around bamboo sticks for shipping

BUFF/BUFFED **1)** To dilute a drug **2)** Muscular in appearance from use of steroids and/or exercise

BUG Itching sensation, due to cocaine overdose

BUGGER Black Tar Heroin

BULLET **1)** Bullet-shaped plastic tube used for snorting drugs in the powdered form **2)** One year jail term

BUMMED/BUMMER **1)** Bad trip **2)** A bad experience not necessarily drug related

BUMP (aka: LINE) **1)** Refers to a line, a bump or pile of cocaine, meth, MDMA or ketamine powder to be snorted, usually 0.2 grams per line **2)** Internet jargon on message boards for agreeing with the last person/message

BUM TRIP A bad hallucinogenic drug experience

BUNK Low grade drug. Often the adulterant is solo and being represented as the drug

BURN   Substances used to dilute potency of drug such as lidocaine, procaine, nicotinamide, or ephedrine

BURNED   Cheated by a drug dealer

BURNED OUT   In a state of brain or chronic behavior impairment resulting from chronic heavy drug use.

BUSH   Marijuana

BUSINESSMAN'S LUNCH   DMT, a hallucinogen with potent effects lasting 30-60 minutes

BUST   An arrest by authorities and confiscation of drugs

BUTTON   The top middle flower area of the Peyote Cactus (Hemispheric Taberculous). A hard, round object, slightly larger than a golf ball, containing the active ingredient of the plant, Mescaline, a hallucinogen

BUTYL NITRATE   A chemical abused by inhalation for the intense rush it provides; was sold over the counter in small vials as incense, cleaner, etc.; may still be diverted from legitimate chemical use

BUY   A drug purchase

BUZZ   A drug high

BZP   In medical notes may refer to benzodiazepine but in the street refers to BENZYLPIPERAZINE, another drug abused by MDMA users for the related effects (See also TFMPP or MOLLY)

C   Cocaine

C&H   Cocaine and Heroin

CABALLO   Spanish word for Heroin

CACTUS   Peyote Cactus

CADET   First time drug user

CALIFORNIA SUNSHINE   LSD produced and sold on the West Coast

CAMEL   Drug smuggler or drug carrier

CAN   One ounce quantity of Marijuana

CANDY   Cocaine or MDMA

CANDY FLIP   Refers to the polydrug "flip" of taking both MDMA and LSD; users are encouraged to take the LSD about three hours before taking Ecstasy (See FLIP)

CANDY MAN   Drug dealer or drug supplier

CANDY RAVER   Rave attendee who dresses in infantile garb, wears bead/candy necklaces and pacifiers and takes the drug MDMA (Ecstasy) (See RAVE)

CAP   1) Powdered drug in capsule form 2) GHB users typically dose in caps, measured by water bottle caps, for example, which is about 6-7ml

CAP-UP   To put powdered drugs into capsules

CARGA   Spanish word for Heroin

CARRIER   Drug smuggler or transporter

CARTWHEELS   White Amphetamine tablets

CAT FOOD   4-methylmethcathinone (See MEPHEDRONE)

CAT **1)** Heroin **2)** A synthetic designer drug, methcathinone, a stimulant with no medical application

CAT VALIUM The drug ketamine, primarily used as a small animal anesthetic but also has use in pediatrics and as a battlefield anesthetic

CATHINONE and CATHINE The leaves of the Khat (or catha edulis) plant common to locations such as Somolia, often chewed for the stimulant effect; when fresh, the leaves contain cathinone, a Schedule I substance, but once dried, the substance deteriorates to the weaker version, cathine, which is on Schedule IV

CCC Refers to the brand "Coricidin Cough & Cold" tablets containing dextromethorphan (DXM), widely abused by teens who take from 10 to 45 pills at a time (See also RED DEVILS, TRIPLE C, THE MATRIX, DXM)

CECIL/CEC Cocaine

CHANNEL Vein used for injecting drugs

CENT One dollar

CHAPAPOTE Spanish word for Mexican Tar Heroin

CHARAS Hindu for Marijuana

CHARGE The first effect of a drug high

CHARLIE Cocaine

CHASING THE DRAGON Heating Heroin or Opium on a piece of foil and inhaling the smoke

CHEESE "Starter heroin" made by mixing ground up Tylenol PM© or Benadryl© (both contain diphenhydramine, an antihistamine with sedating properties) tablets with up to approximately 8 percent of heroin to introduce teens to taking heroin. Mostly in the Dallas, Texas, area (also seen as Chees, Cheez, Chez, Chz, Queso, Keso, Kso in text and email messages)

CHINA WHITE **1)** Southeastern Asian Heroin **2)** The synthetic opiate Alpha-Methylfentanyl

CHIPPER/TO CHIP **1)** An occasional drug user **2)** To inject just under the skin

CHIPPING Taking narcotic analgesics on an occasional or irregular basis, not sufficiently often enough to become physically dependent

CHIVA Spanish word for Heroin

CHOKING GAME A method of self-asphyxiation by cutting off the supply of oxygen/blood flow to the brain by pressing the thumbs against the carotid artery for the high or rush it gives and causing the person to pass out briefly, fall limp and thus release the flow of blood; this game has been around for years but has reached higher risk levels by involving others as the choker and utilizing belts or other props, increasing the risk that airflow or blood flow would be withheld too long, causing brain damage or death; participants are often young teens

CHOPPING To dilute or adulterate a drug

CHRISTMAS TREES The prescription drug Tuinal

CHRONIC High grade marijuana

CIRCLES Rohypnol

CLEAN Drug free

CLENBUTEROL   Abused by some bodybuilders/athletes for alleged fat burning, stimulant and muscle enhancing effects, despite negative side effects

CLUB DRUGS   Common term for a variety of drugs used in rave and nightclub scene, loosely including MDMA (Ecstasy), LSD, ketamine, GHB, meth, marijuana and other hallucinogens

CLUCK HEAD   Street gang term for Cocaine addict

COASTING   The euphoric high just after taking a drug, usually associated with Heroin

COAST TO COASTS   Amphetamine tablets

COCAINE BLUES   Depression from discontinuing use of cocaine

COKE   Cocaine

COKE BUGS   The sensation of bugs crawling under or on the user's skin associated with a Cocaine overdose

COKE HEAD   A Cocaine user

COKE SPOON   A small metal spoon used for snorting (inhaling) Cocaine

COKED OUT   Excessive use of cocaine to point of incoherence

COKED UP   Label for erratic behavior due to excessive use of cocaine

COLA   Cocaine

COLD TURKEY   Abrupt withdrawal from long term drug abuse

COLUM   Street gang term used for Colombian Marijuana

COME DOWN   The gradual wearing-off of the effects of drugs

COME-ON   The first feeling after taking a drug

COMMERCIAL   Street gang term used for Marijuana

CONNECT/CONNECTION   Drug dealer or supplier

CONTACT HIGH   Mild euphoria occurring in non-smokers and believed by them to be the result of inhalation of the Marijuana fumes produced by smokers

COOK   To prepare or heat a drug into liquid form in preparation for injection

COOKED   High on drugs

COOKER   1) The container in which drugs are heated for injection. For example: Spoons, bottle caps, bottom half of a soft drink or beer can, etc. 2) One who manufactures drugs in a lab

COOKIE   Chunk of rock cocaine

COOKING COTTONS   When a Heroin addict can not get Heroin, he will use the old cotton

COP   To purchase drugs

CO-PILOT   An individual knowledgeable about the effects of hallucinogens, particularly in the case of LSD The Co-Pilot provides reassurance and reality for the novice user (See BABYSITTER)

CORINE   Cocaine

COTTON   A small amount of cotton used to filter impurities from dissolved Heroin as it is drawn into the hypodermic

COTTON, ASKING FOR   Refers to an impoverished heroin addict to afford a "buy" scrounging the cotton used as a filter by other addicts that a very weak heroin solution can be made

COTTON FEVER   During the process of injecting, a small piece of cotton is used as a filter when the drug, usually Heroin, is drawn up into the syringe. Occasionally a fiber of cotton is drawn up into the syringe and is injected causing the user to become extremely ill

COTTON MOUTH   Dry mouth caused by ingestion of certain drugs

COURIER   Drug smuggler or transporter

CRACK   Cocaine Hydrochloride (powder) that has been processed into a pure solid form for smoking

CRACK HOUSE   A structure where Crack (Freebased Cocaine) is sold

CRACKER   A device used to "crack open" small nitrous oxide cartridges and divert the gas into a balloon for huffing (See NITROUS OXIDE or WHIPPETS)

CRANK   Methamphetamine

CRANKSTER   User of Methamphetamine

CRANK BUGS   The sensation of bugs crawling on or under the user's skin associated with a Methamphetamine overdose

CRAP   1) Heroin 2) Low quality drug

CRASH   To abruptly stop using a drug

CRATE   A large quantity of pills, usually 50,000

CRATER   A deep flesh indentation at a particular site which has been subjected to repeated intravenous injections

CRINK   Methamphetamine

CROKE   To use Cocaine and Methamphetamine together

CROSS-TOPS   Benzedrine tablets, so named for the crossed lines on one side of the pill as a result of the pill press mold.

CRYSTAL   Methamphetamine

CUBE   A sugar cube containing LSD

CUT   To adulterate or dilute drugs

CYCLING   Using different types of steroids one after another, but not at the same time. Example: Use a particular type of steroid for a period of time then use a different type of steroid to gain the maximum effect and reduce side effects

D   LSD

D & G   MDMA pills with the logo D&G for clothing designers Dolce & Gabanna, one of many business logos used on the illicit pills

DANCE   Refers to the drug carisoprodol (tradename Soma)

DANCING   Mixing the effects of carisoprodol (Soma) with alcohol

DATE RAPE DRUG (RAPE DRUG)   Any drug used to render someone unable to give or withhold consent to sexual activity, such as CNS depressants or hallucinogens (See DFSA)

DATURA   The genus of plants commonly called jimson weed, angel's trumpet, moonflower, devil's weed; leaves, seeds and roots contain atropine, scopolamine and hyoscyamine, three toxic alkaloids; abuse by smoking or making tea to hallucinate can be fatal

DAVA   Heroin

DAZZLE   The depressant drug midazolam (tradename Versed) which is from the family of benzodiazepines

DEAD PRESIDENTS   Street gang term for money

DEAL/DEALER   To sell drugs/One who sells drugs

DEATH   Refers to the drugs PMA and PMMA, similar to MDMA but more intense in effects and have a greater risk of death

DESIGNATED SITTER   Someone who babysits others who are tripping on hallucinogens

DESIGNER DRUG   Drugs designed by chemists as similar to the chemistry and property of other drugs, often to try to sidestep the law if the primary drug is already illegal. Also loosely used interchangeably by some with the term Club Drugs (See ANALOG)

DEVIL DUST   PCP

DEXIES   The prescription stimulant drug Dexedrine

DFSA or DRUG FACILITATED SEXUAL ASSAULT   The use of drugs to render a person unable to give or withhold consent to have sex (See DATE RAPE DRUG)

DIAMONDS   Amphetamine tablets

DILLIES   Dilaudid (Hydromorphine)

DIME   Ten dollars

DIME BAG   Ten dollars worth of a drug

DIRTY   1) To possess drugs 2) To give a positive body fluid test

DIRTY PEE   Positive urine test

DITCH WEED   Low quality Marijuana

D.M.T.   The synthetic hallucinogen Dimethyltryptamine, also called "Businessman's lunch because the effects last less than an hour

DO A LINE   To snort (inhale) a "line" of a drug in powder form

DOING CAPS   Taking GHB by the capful

DO UP   To inject

D.O.A.   Dead on arrival

DOB   2,5 dimethyoxy-4-bromoamphetamine, potent hallucinogen, one of many that may be encountered as a substitute for MDMA

DOLLAR   One hundred dollars worth of a drug

DOLLY   Dolophine (Methadone)

DOOBIE   Marijuana cigarette (See JOINT)

DOORS & FOURS   Taking the prescription drugs Doriden and Tylenol w/Codeine #4 together. The effects are similar to that of Heroin

DOPE   General term for drugs

DOPE FIEND   Drug user

DOPER   Drug user

DOSE   1) The amount of a drug taken 2) The amount of Methadone, a synthetic narcotic used to treat Heroin addiction, that is taken

DOSING   Taking drugs

DOT   A dose of LSD so small it is hard to see

DOUBLE STACK   An MDMA (Ecstasy) pill that is double thick in size and dosage; also a nickname for the deadly drug PMA that is similar to MDMA but more severe

DOWNER   Barbiturates or tranquilizers

DOWN, GET DOWN   Inject a drug

DRAGGED   A mild anxiety and fatigue state following Marijuana intoxication

DREAMERS   Narcotic analgesic drugs

DRIVERS   The prescription drug Benzedrine, however, it is no longer manufactured (See BENNIES and BENZ)

DRONE   4-methylmethcathinone (See MEPHEDRONE)

DROP   To take a drug orally

DROP A TAB   To take LSD orally

DROP A DIME   To inform on someone

DROPPER   Hypodermic syringe

DRUGGIE   Drug user

DRY   1) To be drug free 2) When the supply of drugs are low or gone

DRY OUT   To abstain from drugs or alcohol after a prolonged use, to the point of substantial or complete loss of tolerance

DRY UP   When drugs, usually narcotics, are not available

DUCKETS   Street gang term for money

DUST   1) A drug in powder form 2) Cocaine 3) PCP (Phencyclidine)

DUST OFF   A commercial air cleaner for computers, etc., that is being abused as an inhalant (See DUSTING)

DUSTED   Under the influence of PCP

DUSTER   PCP user

DUSTING   1) Combining marijuana and heroin and rolling it in a form to be smoked 2) Inhaling the spray product DUST OFF

DXM   The cough suppressant dextromethorphan, commonly abused especially by teens; taken in quantities from 300 to 900 milligrams to achieve high and/or hallucinations

DYNO   High quality drug

EASY LAY   The drug gamma hydroxybutyrate, GHB

EAT   To swallow drugs rather than be caught with them

ECHOES   LSD flashbacks

ECSTACY   Refers to ephedrine and herbal products seeking to resemble the drug MDMA in terms of stimulating effects. Note the spelling difference from the drug MDMA's nickname ECSTA_S_Y

E/ECSTASY   The synthetic drug MDMA (3,4-Methylenedioxy-N-Methylamphetamine); See also XTC or X

EIGHT BALL   1/8 ounce of a drug

EIGHTH   1/8 of an ounce or a gram

ELEPHANT   PCP (Phencyclidine)

ELEPHANT FLIP   The polydrug flip of PCP and MDMA

ELEVEN-FIVE-FIFTY   Under the influence of a controlled substance California Health & Safety Code section violation (11550 H&S)

EMBALMING FLUID   An old nickname for PCP but current use also involves the actual abuse of embalming fluid, which contains formaldehyde and gives a similar bizarre behavior state but without the analgesic effect of pain blocking (see PCP, FRY CIGARETTES, ILLY)

EMERALD TRIANGLE   The California counties of Mendocino, Humbolt, and Trinity. This area is know for growing the high grade Sinsemilla Marijuana

EQUIPMENT   Drug paraphernalia

E-PRESSED   Slang for the after effects of MDMA (Ecstasy) depression due to the draining of serotonin levels by this drug

E PUDDLE   Refers to MDMA (Ecstasy) abusers as they often pile up together due to fatigue and/or the general effects of the drug; also called a Cuddle Puddle

EQUIPOISE   A veterinary steroid product, commonly diverted and abused by steroid users, that contains boldenone undecylenate

E-TARD   Someone on MDMA, Ecstasy

E-TARDATION   The "dumbing down" effects of abusing the drug MDMA

EUPHORIA or U4EUH   Hallucinogen 4-methylaminorex

EVERCLEAR   **1)** 190 proof grain alcohol **2)** slang for gamma hydroxybutyrate (GHB)

EYE CANDY   Refers to flashing lights and toys that captivate people who are on the drug MDMA

EYE OPENER   The first Heroin injection of the day

FACTORY   A location where illicit drugs are produced for street sale

FANTASIA   Dimethyltryptamine or DMT

FANTASY   Gamma hydroxybutyrate (GHB) nickname common in Australia where is has been widely abused by bodybuilders and raver/club attendees

FENTANYL   A powerful anesthetic drug. Fentanyl may be diverted from hospitals for use. Analogs of fentanyl are usually manufactured illegally in clandestine drug labs

FINGER   An amount of Marijuana or Hashish

FIRE A LINE   To snort (inhale) an amount of a powdered drug

FIRE UP   To light and smoke a Cocaine or Methamphetamine pipe

FIRE WATER   A GBL product sold as a dietary supplement but now illegal as a GHB analog

FIRED UP   A drug high usually associated with Cocaine or Methamphetamine

FIT   Paraphernalia for injecting drugs

FIVE CENTS   Five dollars worth of a drug

FIX   To inject a drug

FLAKE   Cocaine

FLAKY   Acting crazy

FLASH/FLASHING   The first effect of a drug

STREET SLANG GLOSSARY

FLASHBACK A reoccurrence of a drug usually associated with LSD or PCP. The drug is stored in the fat cells and may reenter the body months or even years after the last ingestion

FLASH POWDER Methamphetamine

FLATLINERS Street drug 4-methylthioamphetamine (4-MTA), also called Golden Eagle

FLIP Polydrug abuse referring to taking, or "flipping" MDMA with other drugs for variation of effects (See CANDY FLIP, HIPPIE FLIP, ELEPHANT FLIP, SEXTASY, LUCKY FLIP)

FLIP OUT To experience a severe psychological reaction to a drug

FLOATING Intoxicated

FLOWER OF PARADISE Refers to khat, a plant often abused in Ethiopian, Somali and Yemeni communities. (See "Cathinone" in stimulant section)

FLUFFING Chopping up Cocaine with a razor blade into a fine powder. It is then strained through mesh to increase its volume

FLYING SAUCER Trade name for Morning Glory seeds

FOILING Placing a drug, usually Heroin, on a piece of tin foil, then heating it up and inhaling the smoke

FOURS 60 mg. Codeine tablets stamped with the number 4

FOXY or FOXY METHOXY Street drug 5-methoxy-N,N-diisopropyltryptamine (5-MEO-DIPT), usually seen in pills with a spider or alien imprint

FREAK One who chronically uses large amounts of a specific drug

FREEBASE or FREEBASING A style of smoking rock cocaine

FREEZE 1)Unavailability of drugs 2) Numbness caused by using cocaine

FRIED 1) Drug high 2) Close to an overdose

FRONT 1)To acquire drugs when payment is to be made by a reliable third party known to the seller 2) To purchase drugs on a short term credit

FRUIT SALAD A reckless combination of drugs

FRY CIGARETTES or FRY STICKS Regular cigarettes or marijuana cigarettes dipped in PCP and/or embalming fluid (See PCP, EMBALMING FLUID & WETS)

GANJA Hindu for Marijuana. Also used in the Jamaican culture

GAP To yawn (one of the earliest symptoms of heroin withdrawal)

GARBAGE Low grade drugs

GBL Gamma butyrolactone, primary ingredient for GHB and an active analog that turns rapidly into GHB in the human body. GBL is a degreasing solvent (See ANALOG)

GEE Gasket between needle and syringe

GEED UP or JEED UP or G'D UP High on gamma hydroxybutyrate (GHB)

GEEZE To inject a drug

GET DOWN To use drugs, but is usually associated with Heroin

GET OFF The first effects of a drug

GHB   Gamma hydroxybutyric acid (like liquid ecstasy). Illegal in U.S. except for limited prescription use under the tradename Xyrem (federal Schedule III drug). If Xyrem is diverted for abuse, it is treated as a Schedule I drug, the same as illicit GHB

GINA   Common gym name for gamma hydroxybutyrate (GHB)

GIRL   Cocaine

GLASS   Pure, solid, smokable form of Crystal Methamphetamine (See ICE)

GOD'S MEDICINE   Morphine

GO/GO FAST   Outdated term for stimulant drugs, usually associated with Amphetamines

GOLD   A particularly potent form of Marijuana grown in the Acapulco area (See ACAPULCO GOLD and GOLD LEAF)

GOLD DUST   Cocaine

GOLDEN CRESCENT   The Opium producing area of Southwest Asia (Iran, Pakistan, and Afghanistan)

GOLDEN TRIANGLE   The Opium producing area of Southeast Asia (Burma, Laos, and Thailand)

GOLD LEAF   A particularly potent form of Marijuana grown in the Acapulco area (See ACAPULCO GOLD and GOLD)

GOMA   Spanish word for Mexican Tar Heroin

GOODS   Refers to narcotics

GOOFBALLS   Barbiturates

GRAM   Common amount or measurement of a drug

GRASS   Marijuana

GRAVEL   Crack Cocaine

GRIFA   Spanish word for Marijuana

GYM CANDY   Street term for anabolic steroid

GUIDE   A baby sitter for an abuser of hallucinogenic drugs during an experience

GUN   Injection paraphernalia H Heroin

HABIT   Drug addiction

HALF   1/2 gram or 1/2 ounce of a drug

HALLUCINOGEN   Also referred to as psychedelic drugs, these substances may be either natural or synthetic and produce various intensities of hallucinations (perceptual changes involving sound, sight, sense of touch or smell, etc.)

HAMMER COMING DOWN   The rapid and dramatic transition from a normal feeling state to that which results from a full impact of a drug. Usually in reference to the effects of a drug intravenously administered

HARD DRUGS   Narcotic analgesics. Also used to cover any drug which is controlled by a federal narcotic statutes, such as cannabis or cocaine

HANYAK   Solid, smokable Methamphetamine

HAPPY DRUG or HAPPY PILL   The drug MDMA

HAPPY DUST   Cocaine

HARD STUFF   Heroin

HASH   The isolated active ingredient of the Marijuana plant, THC; Hash comes in solid and oil form

HAY   Marijuana

HEAD   A heavy regular user of a drug. Reference is often made to a specific drug, such as "Acid Head"

HEAD SHOP   A store that sells drug paraphernalia and other related drug items

HEARTS   Dexedrine tablets

HEAVENLY BLUE   Strain of blue Morning Glory seeds which can be abused by sucking large quantities or making tea from them. Legend is that the blue ones are more potent.

HEAVES   Violent vomiting occurring during drug withdrawal

HEMP   Marijuana

HERB   Marijuana

HIERBA   Street name (Spanish) for marijuana

HIGH   Drug induced euphoria

HIPPIE or HIPPY FLIP   Polydrug flip of MDMA and magic mushrooms

HIT   1) Injection of drugs 2) A puff of a Marijuana Cigarette

HIT UP   1) To inject a drug 2) To borrow or attempt to borrow

HOG   PCP (Phencyclidine)

HOLDING   To possess drugs

HONEY OIL   Purified Hashish Oil containing the highest concentration of THC

HOOKA   Marijuana smoking pipe or bong (See BONG)

HOOKED   Addicted to drugs

HORN   To snort (inhale) drugs in powder form

HORSE   Heroin

HOT SHOT   A very pure dose of Heroin which can result in death

HOUSEWIFE'S DISEASE   Dependence on tranquilizers

HUBBA   Cocaine Freebase

HUFFER   A person who uses inhalants such as glue, paint thinner, petroleum products, etc

HUFFING   The act of using inhalants

HUG DRUG   MDMA (Ecstasy)

HUNTING   Desperately seeking drugs prior to the onset of withdrawal

HUSTLING   Addicts attempts to obtain enough money to purchase more drugs

HYPE   Heroin addict

ICE   Pure, solid, smokable form of Crystal Methamphetamine (See GLASS). Also refers to 4-methylaminorex, which is often called Euphoria or U4EUH.

ILLY CIGARETTE or ILLIES   Regular cigarettes or marijuana cigarettes dipped in PCP and/or embalming fluid (See EMBALMING FLUID, WETS, FRYS)

J Marijuana

JAB To inject

JACKING OFF THE NEEDLE After putting the needle into the vein, some users pull the needle in and out of the wound to be sure the needle is still in the vein. This is usually associated with Heroin use

JAG State of being under influence of solvents

JANE Marijuana

JAR 100 or 1000 pills, also known as jug

JELLY Cocaine

JENKEM Fecal matter & urine are fermented; the gas is captured in a balloon and then inhaled for a brief high. Allegedly done in poverty areas in some countries. Not likely widely practiced anywhere

JET FUEL PCP

JIB Street name for gamma hydroxybutyrate (GHB)

JIM JONES Street gang term for Marijuana cigarette laced with Cocaine and dipped in PCP

JIMSON WEED A hallucinogenic weed from the Datura genus (See DATURA)

JOINT Marijuana cigarette

JOLT The first effects of a drug

JONES A drug habit

JOY POP Irregular use of narcotics

JONESING Needing a drug fix

JOY POPPING To inject just under the skin usually associated with Heroin use

JUG 1,000 pills

JUICE 1) Cheap wine 2) More recently, liquid preparations of narcotic analgesic cough suppressants 3) PCP (Phencyclidine) 4) steroids 5) GHB

JUNK Diluted Heroin

JUNKIE Drug addict

JUNK WEED Low grade Marijuana

K Kilogram (2.2 pounds)

K or KET Ketamine

K2 Herbal mixtures combined with synthetic cannabinoids or cannabinoid-mimicking compounds such as HU-210 and JWH-018 have been surfacing worldwide in a variety of products also referred to by various names, including Spice, Genie, Skunk and Sense. (See SPICE)

KAKSONJAE Pure, solid, smokable form of Crystal Methamphetamine

KAVA KAVA Sold as a dietary supplement, kava is a root common to the South Pacific, containing piper methysticum, that is a mild depressant

KETAMINE Animal tranquilizer for small animals, especially cats, that is also used on a limited basis in humans (in pediatrics and as a war zone anesthetic)

K-HOLE A ketamine induced out of body and/or comatose state

KIBBLES & BITS Street gang term for small pieces of freebase cocaine

KEG 50,000 pills

KEESTER PLANT Drugs which are hidden in the rectum

KGB (KILLER GREEN BUD) Marijuana

KHAT A plant common to areas like Somolia; leaves are chewed for stimulant effect of cathinone (when leaves are fresh) or cathine (once dried) (See CATHINONE and CATHINE)

KICK Stop using drugs

KILLER JOINT or KILLER WEED **1)** Marijuana cigarette laced with PCP **2)** Very potent Marijuana

KILO Kilogram (2.2 pounds)

KINGS HABIT The use of Cocaine

KIT Paraphernalia for injecting drugs

KITTY FLIP The polydrug abuse of using MDMA and ketamine together; abusers are advised to take the MDMA 15 minutes before taking the ketamine (See FLIP)

KJ PCP saturated menthol cigarette (See KOOL JOINT)

KNOCKOUT DRUGS Liquid Chloral Hydrate or other drug, typically used with alcohol, to facilitate rape or robbery; Additional Comments: Despite the terminology, not all drugs used to facilitate rape result in being unconscious. Amnesia is the primary effect for many of them and unconsciousness may or may not occur at some point

KONA GOLD High grade Hawaiian Marijuana

KOOL JOINT Menthol cigarette laced with PCP (See KJ)

KRATOM Unregulated recreational herbal plant increasingly being used for stimulating effects in low doses or opiate, sedating effects in higher doses

KRYSTAL Crystal Methamphetamine

L LSD

LACE To add a drug to another substance. Example: To spray PCP on Marijuana for smoking

LACTONE Gammabutyrolactone (GBL), which is the primary ingredient in GHB but also an active analog; if consumed, GBL converts rapidly in the body to GHB

LADY Cocaine

LAUGHING GAS Nitrous oxide, used legitimately by dentists mixed with controlled level of oxygen but abused by huffing for the brief high that may result in brief unconsciousness (See NITROUS OXIDE)

L.A. TURNAROUNDS Amphetamines

L.B. 1 pound of a drug

LEAF Marijuana

LEAPERS Amphetamines

LEB Lebanese Hashish

LIBS The prescription drug Librium

LID An ounce of marijuana

LIGHT UP To smoke marijuana

LINE An amount of powdered drugs such as cocaine, meth, MDMA or ketamine that is combed (with a credit card or razor) into thin lines (on a mirror or glass or smooth surface) for snorting (with a straw or rolled up paper currency, etc.) (See BUMP)

LIQUID XTC or LIQUID X or LIQUID ECSTASY Refers to the drug GHB which is most commonly found in liquid state; does not refer to MDMA (Ecstasy) though some abusers have accidentally taken it believing it is a liquid version of MDMA

LOADED Under the influence of a drug

LOADS Tylenol® w/ Codeine® #4 and Doriden®

LOCO WEED Marijuana

LOVE DRUGS MDA, Methqualone

LOVE FLIP Polydrug abuse of MDMA and Mescaline

LOVELY PCP

LSA d-lysergic acid amide is a precursor chemical to LSD and can be derived by sucking on morning glory seeds or drinking tea made from the seeds

LSD The synthetic hallucinogen D-Lysergic Acid Diethylamide

LUCKY FLIP Polydrug abuse of MDMA and Lucky 7 (2-CT-7)

LUCKY 7 Street drug 2C-T-7, also called Triptasy, T7, 7-UP and Blue Mystic (See TRYPTAMINE)

LUDES Quaaludes (No longer manufactured)

M 1) Marijuana 2) Morphine

M&M's MDMA (3,4-Methylenedioxyl-N-Methylamphetamine)

MAGIC DUST PCP

MAGIC MUSHROOM Refers to Psilocybin

MAKE A BUY Purchase drugs

MAINLINE To inject intravenously

MAN Drug dealer or drug connection

MANICURE The removal of unusable parts of the Marijuana plant such as stocks, stems, seeds, etc

MANNITOL Cutter for cocaine

MAPS The Multidisciplinary Association for Psychedelic Studies is a nonprofit group that promotes research of all psychedelic drugs and promotes legalization

MARKS Puncture wounds or holes left from needle injection

MARKED UP Displaying puncture wounds from needle injections

MARY JANE Marijuana

MATCHBOX 1/2 ounce of marijuana

MAUI WOWIE High grade Marijuana from Hawaii

STREET SLANG GLOSSARY

MDA   Mellow Drug of America. The synthetic hallucinogen drug 3,4-Methylenedioxyamphetamine

MDMA   3,4-Methylenedioxy-N-Methylamphetamine is a synthetic hallucinogen with stimulant qualities

MEOW-MEOW   4-methylmethcathinone (See MEPHEDRONE)

MEPHEDRONE   Marketed on the Internet as a "plant food," mephedrone is 4-methylmethcathinone (4-MMC). It is a stimulant with some psychotropic effects much like MDMA (Ecstasy). It is also known as drone, bubble or bubbles, meow meow, MM-Cat, M-Cat, cat food, and Sunshine

MEQUIN   Methaqualone

MERCK   Pharmaceutical Cocaine

MERSH   Low grade Marijuana

MESC   Mescaline

METH   Methamphetamine

METH MOUTH   Deterioration of the teeth from exposure to the chemicals involved in methamphetamine and drug's effect of causing mouth dryness

METHADONE   Methadone is most commonly known for use in heroin addiction treatment; it is also a pain medication being more widely prescribed, resulting in increased abuse and deaths

METHCATHINONE   A street drug stimulant related to meth and often called CAT

METH HEAD   User of methamphetamine

MEXICAN BROWN   Mexican brown heroin

MEXICAN MUD   Mexican black tar heroin

MICKEY FINN   The combination of the prescription drug Chloral Hydrate and Alcohol

MICRO DOTS   LSD on very small tablets

MIERA   Spanish word for Heroin

MIKE   Microgram

MILK   From milk sugar. Crystals of lactose frequently used in diluting Heroin

MIND-BLOWING   Referring to a drug that produces extraordinarily powerful reaction. Usually a favorable experience

MINI BEANS   Small Benzedrine tablets

MISS EMMA   Morphine

MITSUBISHI   MDMA pill with the Mitsubishi corporate logo imprinted; pill may be round, triangular or pentagon shaped; a very common logo

MJ   Marijuana

MMDA   3-Methoxy-4, 5 Methylenedioxyamphetamine which is a psychedelic Amphetamine

MOLLY   The drug TFMPP or 1-(3-Trifluoromethylphenyl) piperazine is referred to as Molly and is typically in capsule form; same clientele as MDMA and similar effects

MONKEY   The state of being in withdrawal from Heroin MOTA Spanish word for Marijuana

MOUTH HABIT   Oral drug use

MPPP   One of the numerous, so called "Designer Drugs" similar to MPTP. Gives Heroin-like effects and can be made to look like White Heroin

MPTP   Made from MPPP and is another "Designer Drug" with effects like White Heroin

MSM   Methyl sulfone or methylsulfoylmethane is a naturally occurring organic sulfur compound, sold as a dietary supplement; also used as a cutting agent for meth; extends quantity and gives a whiter product

MUD   Mexican black tar heroin

MULE   A drug smuggler who actually carries the drugs

MUNCHIES   Constant snacking associated with Marijuana intoxication

MUSCLING   Injecting drugs into the muscle and is most commonly associated with steroids

NAIL   Hypodermic needle

NARC   1) A narcotics officer 2) An informer 3) To inform on someone, "To narc someone off"

NEBBIES   The prescription drug Nembutal

NEEDLE FREAK   One who injects drugs into the vein or skin

NEEDLE MAN   An addict

NEXUS   The drug 2-(4-Bromo-2,5-dimethoxy-phenyl)-ethylamine, also called 2C-B or Bromo

NEXUS FLIPPING   Taking MDMA and Nexus (See FLIP)

NICKEL   Five dollars

NICKEL BAG   Five dollars worth of a drug

NINETEEN   A term for speed. The nineteenth letter of the alphabet is "S"

NOD   Being under the influence of Heroin. A relaxed state similar to sleep

NOSE CANDY   Cocaine

NOX   Abusing nitrous oxide while on MDMA

NOZ   Reference to nitrous oxide

N2O   Nitrous oxide, abused by inhaling, causing a very brief high and possible brief unconsciousness; not scheduled but some states have laws against possession with intent to inhale (gas, devices for inhaling, etc.) and for inhaling or being impaired to drive

NUBAIN   Brand name for the drug nalbuphine, an analgesic for moderate to severe pain; widely used by athletes, often resulting in abuse and addiction

NUKING THE COKE   During the Cocaine Freebasing process the Cocaine Hydrochloride is mixed with baking soda and water, then heated. The microwave is used to speed up the process. A coffee maker machine may also be used

NUTMEG   Cooking herb abused by some in high quantities (5-20 grams) for hallucinogenic effects; contains myristicin (also contained in mace)

O   **1)** Cocaine **2)** Opium

O.D.   Overdose, usually a very serious condition

OCOTEA   Ocotea Cymbarum, distilled from the bark of trees native to Brazil, Paraguay and Colombia and containing safrole, a key precursor for making MDMA; also called Oil of Octea and Brazilian sassafras oil

OIL   **1)** Hashish in oil form **2)** Methamphetamine in oil form

OLLA   Cocaine

ONE HITTER   A drug that can only be diluted one time

ONE & ONE   Two lines of Cocaine, one for each nostril

ON THE PIPE   Street gang term for being addicted to Freebase Cocaine

ORANGE CRUSH   When the red pills of Coridicin® Cough & Cold medication are crushed it results in an orange powder that is then snorted for the high from the DXM it contains (See DXM or DEXTROMETHORPHAN)

OTC   Over the counter. Refers to drugs that can be bought without a prescription

OUTFIT   Paraphernalia for injecting drugs

OUT OF SIGHT   **1)** Extraordinary quality, wonderful **2)** A fantastic experience

OVERAMPED   An overdose usually associated with a stimulant drug (Cocaine or Methamphetamine)

OXY/OXYCOTTON   OxyContin, brandname for the synthetic opiate oxycodone; widely abused for its powerful euphoria but also potentially deadly

OZ/OZER   One ounce

PAKALOLO   Hawaiian for Marijuana

PANAMA GOLD   High grade Panamanian Marijuana

PANAMA RED   High grade Panamanian Marijuana that has a red color to the leaves and a red fuzz on the under portion of the leaves

PANIC   **1)** An acute state of fear precipitated by the onset of withdrawl and frantic action to acquire drugs **2)** An abrupt drying up of heroin sources, affecting all local addicts

PAPERS   **1)** Marijuana rolling papers (Zig-Zag being the most common) **2)** Blotter acid **3)** A piece of paper folded like an envelope containing a small amount of a drug (See BINDLE)

PAPER ACID   LSD

PARACHUTE   MDMA powder or crushed MDMA pills or coke powder may be wrapped in tissue and swallowed in the belief that letting the drug "parachute" down in that manner intensifies the effect

PARTY BOWL/PARTY BONG   A Marijuana pipe (See BONG)

PAREST   Methaqualone

PASTA/PASTE   Raw coca extracted from the coca leaves to be refined into Cocaine Hydrochloride. The raw coca is often smoked by the local peasants because of its availability and inexpensive price

PAYS & OWES   Paperwork (may be elaborate bookkeeping or scraps of paper) showing buyers, sales and/or money amounts re drug distribution; may be in code

PCP   Phencyclidine

P.D.R.   Physician's Desk Reference. A book that contains all the pharmaceutical drugs. Used by doctors

PCE   N-Ethyl-1 -Phenycyclhexylamine. An analog or member of the PCP family of drugs

PEACE WEED   Marijuana laced with PCP

PEAKING   Reaching the highest point while under the influence of a drug

PEARL   Cocaine

PEARLS   Amyl Nitrite

PEANUT BUTTER CRANK   Low grade crude Methamphetamine

PEDAZO   Spanish word for Heroin

PEP PILL   Amphetamine

PERCS   The prescription drug Percodan

PERICO   Spanish word for Cocaine

PERSIAN BROWN   Raw, unprocessed Morphine sold on the streets as Heroin

PERSIAN WHITE   High grade Persian Heroin

PERUVIAN FLAKE   South American high grade Cocaine and refers to the shape of the Cocaine crystals

PEYOTL   American Indian name for the Peyote Cactus

PEZ   LSD-laced PEZ candies

PHARMING   The dangerous practice of mixing a variety of prescription and/or over-the-counter medications in a bowl at a party and grabbing a few without regard for dosage and drug interaction; also called TRAIL MIX

PHENETHYLAMINES   A class of chemical compounds that produce hallucinogenic effects and varying degrees of stimulation, best known being MDMA, MDA, MDEA, 2-CB

PHENNIES   The prescription drug Phenobarbital

PIECE   1 ounce, or 1 pound, of a drug

PILL FREAK   User of any type of pills

PILLOW   1) Methamphetamine 2) Package of 1,000 Amphetamine tablets 3) Methaqualone

PINNED   Constricted pupils (the size of a pinhead) that result when under the influence of Heroin or other narcotics

PIN/PINNER   A very thin Marijuana cigarette

PINK HEARTS   1) Prescription drug Preludin 2) Fake stimulants that can be ordered out of magazines and contain Caffeine and/or Ephedrine

PINK LADIES   The prescription drug Darvon

PINKS   Seconal (named for the color of the capsule)

STREET SLANG GLOSSARY

PIPERAZINE A veterinary animal wormer; variations of it are abused drugs (See BZP and TFMPP) with stimulant and somewhat MDMA-like properties

PIPERIDINE Used to make PCP

PLATEAUING Peaking out on a drug to the point where the user no longer feels the designated effects. Usually used to describe steroids

PLUGGING The practice of rectal insertion of MDMA pills

PLUR Raver term standing for Peace Love Unity and Respect

POLVO Spanish word for Cocaine

POP 1) To take a tablet orally 2) To inject subcutaneous

POPPERS Amyl and Butyl Nitrite, which is administered by crushing the small vile in which it is contained and immediately inhaling the vapors

POPPING 1) To swallow a drug 2) To inject a drug under the skin, not directly into the vein

POT Marijuana

POT HEAD Marijuana user

POWDERED Under the influence of Cocaine

P-2-P Phenyl-2-Propanone. A chemical used to make methamphetamine

PRIMO Street gang term for a Marijuana cigarette laced with Cocaine

PROCAINE Adulterant used to dilute the strength of cocaine or Mexican brown heroin; has pharmacological action of its own

PROGESTEREX Fake drug touted in email over several years claiming that women are being drug raped and given Protesterex which will render them infertile. There is no such drug

PROP Phenly-2-Propanone. A chemical used for manufacturing methamphetamine

PSYCHEDELIC A drug that distorts visual, auditory, and tactil senses

PUMPERS Street term for anabolic steroid

PUNTA ROJA High grade Columbian Marijuana

PURPLE HEARTS Phenobarbital (Luminal tablets)

PURPLE STICKY Brand name in head shops for Mexican salvia (See SALVIA DIVINORUM)

PUSHER Seller of drugs at the street level

PYRAMIDS Brightly colored gelatin LSD on pieces of diffuser plastic (from fluorescent light fixtures, for example); may be peeled off of the plastic and cut into little strips like modern-day breath mint strips or the plastic may be perforated and then broken into square or rectangular pieces which are sucked on by the user

Q'S Methaqualone

QUARTER 1) 1/4 gram of a drug 2) 1/4 ounce of a drug 3) $25.00 worth of a drug

QUARTER PIECE 1/4 ounce of a certain drug

RACK 2-5 capsules wrapped in tin foil

RAGWEED Low grade Marijuana

RAILS   Lines of a powdered drug laid beside each other, on a mirror or a piece of glass, in preparation for snorting (inhaling)

RAINBOWS   Tuinal (a combination of amobarbital and secobarbital) so called because of the bright red and blue capsules (See RED & BLUES)

RAT   An informer

RAVE PARTY   All night electronic music party where most attendees use hallucinogens, especially MDMA (Ecstasy), and other drugs

REDS/REDEVILS   1) Seconal 2) also refers to the red tablets containing DXM marketed as Coricidin Cough and Cold (See also ROBOTRIPPIN' and DXM)

RED & BLUES   Tuinal. Bright red and blue capsules (See RAINBOWS)

REEFER   A Marijuana cigarette

REGISTER   To find the vein when injecting

RENEWTRIENENT   A common GHB analog product disguised as a dietary supplement but illegal for human consumption; usually contains GBL

RESIN   The active ingredient of the Marijuana plant. THC (Delta-9-Tetrahydrocannabinol)

RIB   Flunitrazepam, also known as Rohypnol

RICIN   A poisonous natural extract isolated from castor beans; falsely claimed to be used by meth traffickers to kill police officers, as per a fake alert that was being distributed via email in recent years

RIG   The paraphernalia used to inject drugs

RIPPED   1) Exhausted after a several day amphetamine run 2) adversely affected by a drug 3) very muscular and lean

RIPPERS   Amphetamines

RIPPED OFF   1) Robbed 2) Cheated in a drug buy

ROACH   The butt end of a Marijuana cigarette

ROACH CLIP   Any object used to hold the last bit of a burning Marijuana cigarette. An electrical alligator clip or surgical hemostat are commonly used

ROACHED OUT   High on flunitrazepam, trade name Rohypnol

ROBOTRIPPIN'   On DXM, named for Robitussin products that contain dextromethorphan, a cough suppressant that causes hallucinations in high doses

ROCA   Spanish word for Crack

ROCK   Freebased Cocaine Hydrochloride

ROCK UP   The process of converting Cocaine Hydrochloride to Cocaine base

ROCKET FUEL   PCP

ROIDS   General term for steroids

ROID RAGE   The uncontrollable, violent temperament displayed by some steroid users

ROLL   10 pills sold in tin foil

ROLLS   MDMA pills

ROLLING or ROLLIN'   On MDMA (Ecstasy)

ROLLER PAPERS   Cigarette rolling papers used to make Marijuana cigarettes

ROMPUM   Horse or large animal tranquilizer, analgesic, and muscle relaxant Xylazine; limited abuse by humans reported for euphoric effect

ROOFIES/ROOPIES   Flunitrazepam, tradename Rohypnol

ROPE   Marijuana

RUBBY   A skid row alcoholic who on occasion resorts to propyl (rubbing) alcohol

RUDERALIS   Russian Marijuana plant. It has a low percentage of THC, the active ingredient in Marijuana

RUFFIES   Flunitrazepam, tradename Rohypnol

RUMMY   Skid row alcoholic

RUN   A period of several consecutive days during which an individual uses Methamphetamines several times a day with little food or sleep

RUNNER   Drug smuggler or transporter

RUSH   An intense sensation which rapidly follows intravenous administration of such drugs as heroin, amphetamines or cocaine

SAFROLE   Key ingredient in MDMA; may appear as iso-safrole, bromo-safrole or chloro-safrole; a sassafras extract but is not present in sassafras candies sold legitimately. No legitimate chemical use in the USA

SALTY WATER   Nickname for GHB. Also referred to as WATER

SALVIA DIVINORUM   A hallucinogenic plant from the mint family that grows wild in some regions of Mexico and used by shamans there; active ingredient is salvinorin A, not scheduled as of 2005. More powerful than marijuana. Being touted on the Internet and in head shops (See PURPLE STICKY)

SATIVA   Marijuana. Comes from the scientific name Cannabis Sativa

SCHOOL BOY   Codeine, so called because of the mildness of its effects when compared with the more potent narcotic analgesics

SCOOP   Common nickname for the drug GHB

SCOPOLAMINE   A Belladonna alkaloid (dispensed in transdermal patches) used to treat motion sickness by reducing nausea. Has been used in drug rape and robbery cases, causing amnesia and drowsiness. One of the three active ingredients in Jimson Weed (aka: ZOMBIE DRUG)

SCORE   To make a successful drug purchase

SCRATCH   Money

SCREENS   Round metal mesh screens placed in a smoking pipe to hold the drug in the bowl

SCRIBE   A person who writes false prescriptions

SCRIPT   Drug prescription

SCRIPT WRITER   Physician willing to write prescriptions for drugs

SECOS   Seconal

SEND IT HOME   To inject narcotic analgesics, cocaine or amphetamines intravenously

SERVE   Street gang term for selling drugs

SES   Sinsemilla Marijuana (Sinsemilla means without seeds)

SET   A combination of the prescription drugs Doriden and Tylenol w/Codeine #4

SET UP   A situation in which undercover police officers entice a person to sell them drugs for the purpose of bringing about the person's arrest

SEXTASY   The "flip" of taking MDMA and Viagra together. The Viagra helps overcome the erectile dysfunction or blockage of orgasms that MDMA may cause

SHABU   Hawaiian word for the smokable form of Crystal Methamphetamine (See GLASS and ICE)

SHAKE   The manicured leaves of a Marijuana plant

SHAVE   **1)** To adulterate, dilute or shortweight a drug **2)** Literally shave off minute quantities and thereby shortweight the buyer

SHEET ACID   LSD on blotter paper (See BLOTTER ACID)

SHERMS   A heavy-stock dark brown paper cigarette that is dipped into PCP and then smoked (Short for Shermans)

SHIT   Low quality drugs usually refers to Heroin

SHOOT-UP   To inject intravenously

SHOOTING GALLERY   A place where heroin addicts congregate to inject

SHORTCHANGED   Having been sold drugs which are usually inferior in quality or purity

SHOTGUNNING   Using any available steroid

SHOT IN THE ARM   Although the general use of the term is now broader, it originally referred to an injection of narcotics, which is followed by a state of peacefulness, reverie and well-being

SHROOMS   The hallucinogenic Psilocybin Mushrooms

SICKNESS   The onset of withdrawal

SINSEMILLA   Spanish for "without seed." Marijuana from unfertilized female plants; it is a method of growing, not a variety of marijuana

SIPPIN' SYRUP   Drinking codeine cough syrup (promoted in a rap song)

SKAG   Heroin

SKIN POPPING   Injecting subcutaneous

SKITTLES or SKITTLING   Refers to being on DXM (See DEXTROMETHORPHAN)

SKUNK WEED   High grade Marijuana with a strong odor

SLAB   A large, flat piece of Freebased cocaine

SLAMMING   To inject. Usually refers to Heroin use

SLEEPERS   Sedative/hypnotic drugs such as barbiturates

SLOW AND LOW   Heroin users, when under the influence are said to be slow and low, in that they move slowly and speak in a low slow, slurred voice

SMACK   Heroin

STREET SLANG GLOSSARY

SMART DRINK   Liquid concoctions containing various amino acids said to increase the intelligence of the user. Common at "rave" parties

SMASHED   Heavily intoxicated with alcohol or other drugs

SMOKE   Marijuana

SMOKE HOUSE   A structure where users go to smoke Freebase Cocaine. They "rent" the pipes which contain the drug and leave the pipe behind

SMURFS   Blue MDMA pills, the color of Smurf cartoon characters

SNAPPERS   Amyl or Butyl Nitrate SNAPS Street gang term for money

SNIFF   1) To take cocaine, amphetamines or heroin by inhaling through the nose 2) To inhale solvents through both the nose and mouth

SNORT   To inhale a drug in powdered form. Usually refers to Cocaine

SNOT   Black Tar Heroin

SNOW   Cocaine

SNOW BIRD   Cocaine

SNOW FLAKE   Cocaine

SNOW BUGS   The sensation of bugs crawling on or under the skin of a Cocaine user

SNOW SEAL   A brand of non-porous smooth paper used to make bindles to carry drugs. Logo is a seal balancing a snowflake on its nose

SOAP   GHB

SOAPER/SOAP   Sopor (Methaqualone)

SODIUM OXYBATE   The drug GHB, tradename Xyrem

SOFT DRUGS   Drugs of abuse other than narcotics also applied to those drugs perceived to have low toxicity and/or dependency liability

SOLES   Slabs of solid Hashish

SOMA   Common street name and a tradename of the abused skeletal muscle relaxant carisoprodol, a depressant

SOURCE   A drug dealer or drug supplier

SPACE BASING   Freebased Cocaine dipped in PCP and then smoked

SPACED   Unresponsive to the external environment, usually in reaction to altered consciousness produced by hallucinogenic drugs

SPACEY   Referring to a strangeness or a state of psychic deterioration produced by excessive and/or heavy, chronic use of drugs

SPEAKER TWEAKER   People high on MDMA who hang onto the speakers at raves for the intense sensation of sound and vibration

SPECIAL K   The drug ketamine

SPEED   Injectable methamphetamine

SPEEDBALL   Heroin plus cocaine

SPEEDFREAK   Heavy regular use of injectable methamphetamine

SPEED LAB   Laboratory where Methamphetamines are manufactured

SPEEDER   Methamphetamine user

SPICE Foil packets with names like Spice, Spice Gold, Spice Silver, Spice Diamond, Genie and Yucatan Fire "incense" test negative by standard marijuana testing, but have been laced with verifiable amounts of synthetic cannabinoids or cannabinoid-mimicking compounds, including HU-210, JWH-018 and other related chemicals. Also known as K2

SPIKE Hypodermic needle

SPOON **1)** Small metal spoon used to snort (inhale) drugs in powdered form **2)** Teaspoon used to heat drugs prior to injection **3)** Street measurement of a drug, usually an amount for personal use and usually refers to Heroin

SPORE The reproductive part of the mushroom

SPORTING Cocaine use

STACKING The use of two or more steroids. One right after another, but not at the same time

STAR DUST Cocaine

STASH **1)** A place where drugs are hidden to escape detection in the event of a sudden search by authorities **2)** To hide drugs rapidly when confronted with a search

STASH CANS Common brand name items, such as beer cans, motor oil cans, in which the bottom or top screws off and the drugs are hidden inside

STEP-ON To dilute a drug

STICK A Marijuana cigarette

STINK WEED Low grade Marijuana

STONED Pleasurably intoxicated

STOOLIE An informant

S.T.P. Serenity, Tranquility, Peace. The synthetic hallucinogen 2,5-Dimethoxy-4-Methlyamphetamine

STRAWBERRY Street gang term for a female who exchanges sex for drugs

STRUNG OUT **1)** In an emaciated and generally poor state of health and appearance due to chronic drug use **2)** Heavily dependent on drugs **3)** Sometimes to produce an extreme negative psychic effect during a single drug episode

STUFF General term for drugs, specifically Heroin

SUGAR (MILK) HABIT Addict's desire for sweets due to heavy amount of milk mixed with everyday heroin

SUNSHINE Long standing term for LSD but also a term for a new drug, methylmethcathinone, which is chemically similar to methcathinone (See methcathinone in stimulant section; see also MEPHEDRONE, MEOW MEOW)

SUPER GRASS **1)** PCP laced Marijuana **2)** High grade potent Marijuana

SUPER JOINT Marijuana cigarette dipped in PCP

SUPER K The prescription drug Ketamine

SUPER WEED **1)** High grade Marijuana **2)** Marijuana laced with PCP

SUPPLIER Drug dealer or drug source

STREET SLANG GLOSSARY

SWEAT IT OUT   To withdraw from narcotic analgesics

SWEEPING   Snorting (inhaling) drugs in powdered form

SWING MAN   A drug supplier

SWIRL or SWIRLING   The drug GHB; the sensation of being on GHB

T   The prescription drug Talwin

T'S AND BLUES   Pentazocine (Talwin) plus tripelennamine prepared in a solution and injected

TABS   LSD

TAKE-OFF   The first effects of a drug

TAR   Mexican black tar heroin

TASTE   Sampling a drug before buying it

TATTOOING   Prior to injecting, some users burn the end of the needle for sterilization. If the carbon deposits that form are not cleaned off prior to injecting, they will form under the skin causing dark marks. Same principle as a standard tattoo

TEA   Marijuana

TEABAGGING   Rectal insertion of tampon soaked in GHB

TEMPLE BALLS   Hashish mixed with Opium then shaped into a small, round ball. Common in Nepal and parts of India

TEN CENTS   Ten dollars

TEN CENT BAG   Ten dollars worth of a drug

TETRAHYDROZOLINE   The active ingredient in Visine© and other eye drop brands; has been used to incapacitate people for purposes of robbery and as a dangerous prank; ingestion can result in blurred vision, lowering of blood pressure, seizures, coma; abusers of GHB and drug rapists often utilize eye drop bottles to hide and transport GHB

TFMPP   The drug TFMPP or 1-(3-Trifluoromethylphenyl) piperazine is referred to as Molly and is typically in capsule form; same clientele as MDMA and similar effects (See MOLLY and BZP)

THAI STICK   Potent Marijuana from Thailand whose buds are attached to six inch sticks with string

THC   Delta 9-Tetrahydrocannabinol. The active ingredient of the Marijuana plant

THE MATRIX   The cough suppressant DXM, referring to the red pill of Coricidin® Cough & Cold and the movie by that name wherein a red pill is taken to enter the matrix

THRUSTERS   Amphetamines

TIE   A tourniquet tied around the arm to inhibit blood flow so the vein will bulge for injecting. Example: Belt, scarf, hose, surgical tubing, etc

TIE UP   To apply a belt or tourniquet to the arm or leg to produce distention of a vein for an injection

TIE RAG   (See TIE)

TIME FLIP   The flip of MDMA and DMT (See FLIP and DMT)

TMA   Trimethoxyamphetamine. Similar to MDA

TOKE   1) A puff of a marijuana cigarette 2) To take a puff

TOKER   Marijuana smoker

TOOLS   Drug paraphernalia

TOOT   Cocaine

TOOTER   A piece of a drinking straw, a rolled up dollar bill, or other device used for snorting (inhaling) powdered drugs

TOPS   The top buds of the Marijuana plant rich in THC

TOTALED   Exhausted after an acute drug experience

TRACKS, TRACK MARKS   **1)** Collapsed veins resulting from chronic injection **2)** discoloration and scars, resembling a tattoo in appearance, resulting from chronic injection

TRAIL MIX   Abuse of multiple prescription drugs and/or over the counter products (See PHARMING)

TRANK   PCP

TRAVELER   A user of hallucinogenic drugs

TREATMENT   A dose of Heroin, especially when feeling the effects of withdrawal

TRIP   Under the influence of a drug. Usually refers to LSD

TRIPPERS   LSD

TRIPLE C   Dextromethorphan (See CCC and DXM)

TRIPLE STACK   An Ecstasy pill three times the normal thickness and dosage

TRYPTAMINES   Class of chemical compounds that produce hallucinogenic effects, most notorious being psilocybin mushrooms, DMT, 2C-T-7, AMT and FOXY

TUIES   The prescription drug Tuinal

TURN ON   **1)** To produce a state of pleasurable excitement (the stimulus may be either a drug or other experience) **2)** To introduce someone to a drug or drugs

TWEAKED   Under the influence of Methamphetamine sometimes refers to an adverse reaction

TWEAKER   Chronic meth abuser at the end of a binge period; dangerous time for confrontation with law enforcement due to high propensity for violence at this stage

UNCUT   A drug that has not been diluted

UP FRONT   **1)** As a sample, a small quantity of a drug is provided to the buyer to indicate quality **2)** As proof, showing the seller the money before the drugs are produced

UPPERS   A general term used for most stimulant drugs of abuse, such as amphetamines, and related drugs. However, the term is not used for cocaine

UP TIGHT   Tense, nervous or frightened because of a subjective experience produced by either a drug or by real events

URINE METH   Saving urine from chronic users to process for the unmetabolized meth

USER   Someone who uses drugs or is an addict

U.S.P.   Pharmaceutical Methamphetamine

VALS   The prescription drug Valium

VAPORS   Gang term for Freebase Cocaine smoke

STREET SLANG GLOSSARY

VEGETABLE   One who suffers from severe brain or behavioral impairment to the point of being unable to care for oneself

VITAMIN K   The drug ketamine (See SPECIAL K)

WACK   1) To dilute or cut a drug 2) PCP

WAFER COCAINE   Rock cocaine in appearance of wafers or pasta style (instead of the typical "rock" format), classic of 18th Street Gang

WAKE-UPS   Amphetamines

WASHBACK   A method used to get any usable drug out of a pipe after it has been used several times (See WASHBACK METHODS)

WASTED   Exhausted after an acute drug experience, usually in reference to amphetamines or cocaine

WATER   1) Methamphetamine 2) GHB

WATER PIPE   A smoking pipe that has a chamber that is filled with water or wine. The chamber is used to cool the smoke (See BONG)

WEDGES   Flat LSD tablets

WEED   1) Marijuana 2) Tobacco

WEEKENDER   An occasional drug user

WET DADDIES   PCP

WETS   Marijuana cigarettes dipped in PCP and/or embalming fluid (See FRYS, PCP, EMBALMING FLUID, ILLY)

WHIP-ITS or WHIPPITS or WHIPPETS   Small nitrous oxide canisters, slightly smaller than CO2 cartridges, used to power whipped cream makers and often abused by inhalation (See CRACKERS, NITROUS OXIDE, N2O)

WHITE   1) Cocaine 2) Asian Heroin

WHITE GIRL   Cocaine

WHITES   Amphetamine tablets

WHITE STUFF   Heroin, usually Chinese

WIGGIN or WIGGING   1) Bizarre behavior on mind-altering drugs 2) in need of drugs 3) on MDMA (Ecstasy)

WINDOW PANE   LSD that is placed on small squares of gelatin

WIPED OUT   To have lost consciousness from abusing drugs

WIRED   1) Chronically dependent on amphetamines 2) Physically dependent on heroin

WIRED-OUT   High on Cocaine or Methamphetamine

WITHDRAW   The effects of quitting the heavy use of narcotics

WORKS   Paraphernalia for injecting drugs

WRECKED   1) Exhausted after an acute drug experience 2) Having a very bad drug experience

X   M.D.M.A.-(3,4-Methylenedioxly-N-Mtheylamphetamine)

XTC   Also known as Ecstacy, MDMA, and Adam. Psychedelic drug common to "rave" parties

YABA   Also called the CRAZY DRUG, YABA is simply pills of meth or a combo of meth/ephedrine; designed to market to teens with the pill format, colors and logos, similar to MDMA marketing

YELLOWS, YELLOW JACKETS   Nembutal (Pentobarbital sodium)

YEN Agitated sleep occurring during withdrawal from heroin Z One ounce of a drug

ZANY BARS The drug alprazolam, tradename Xanax, a benzodiazepine depressant; refers to the format sometimes used for this drug which is bars with marks for breaking off doses as directed

ZIP/ZIPPY Amphetamines

ZOMBIE DRUG See SCOPOLAMINE

ZONKED Extremely high on drugs

This page intentionally left blank.

INDEX

A

Adderall, 110
Adipex, 123
Alcohol, 14
Alfenta, 75
Alfentanyl, 75
Alpha-methyl fentanyl, 75
Alprazolam, 23
Ambien, 28, 29
Amitriptyline HCl, 31
Amobarbital, 17
Amoxapine, 31
Amphetamines, 110
AMT, 41
Amyl/Butyl Nitrite, 67
Amytal, 17
Anafranil, 31
Analgesic, 183
Analog, 183
Anti-Depressants, 31
Apo-Trimip, 31
Aquachloral, 19
Asendin, 31
Atarax, 29
Ataxia, 183
Ativan, 22, 23
Autoerotic Asphyxiation, 164
Aventyl, 31
Avinza, 91

B

Barbiturates, 16
BD, 24, 25, 26, 27
Benadryl, 29
Benzodiazepines, 22
Benzphetamine, 123
benzyl fentanyl, 75
Benzylpiperazine, 59
Black Tar Heroin, 76
Brevital, 17
Bromazepam, 23
Buprenex, 97
Buprenorphine, 97
Bupropion, 31
Businessman's Lunch, 42
BuSpar, 19
Buspirone, 19
Butabarbital Sodium, 17
Butalbital, 16, 17
Butisol, 17
Butorphanol Tartrate, 97

BZP, 59

C

Caffeine, 123
Captagon & Theophylline, 124
Carisoprodol, 19
Cat, 118, 119
Celexa, 31
Centrax, 23
Cheese, 80
China White, 76, 77
Chloral hydrate, 19
Chlordiazepoxide, 23
Chlorpromazine, 21
Choking Game, 164
Citalopram HCl, 31
Clomipramine, 31
Clonazepam, 22, 23
Clorazepate, 23
Clozapine, 21
Clozaril, 21
Cocaine, 112, 114
Cocaine Sifter, 137
Codeine, 72
Compazine, 21
Concerta, 111
Crack, 112
Crank, 116
Cyclohexyl Nitrite, 67
Cylert, 111

D

Dalmane, 23
Damason, 85
Darvocet, 97
Darvon, 97
Datura, 44, 45
Demerol, 87
Desipramine, 31
Desoxyn, 111
Desyrel, 30, 31
Dexedrine, 111
Dexfenfluramine, 123
Dextroamphetamine, 110, 111
Dextromethorphan, 106
Dextrostat, 111
Diacetylmorphine, 76, 77
Diazepam, 22, 23
Didrex, 123
Diethylpropion, 122
Dilaudid, 82
Diphenhydramine HCl, 29

217

Dissociative Anesthetic, 24, 25, 27
D-Lysergic Acid Amide, 48
DMT, 41
Dolophine, 88, 89
Doral, 23
Doriden, 19
Dospan, 123
Doxepin HCl, 31
Droperidol, 21
Duragesic, 75
Duramorph, 91
DXM, 106

E
Effexor, 31
Elavil, 31
Endocet, 95
Endodan, 95
Ephedrine, 123
Equanil, 19
Escitalopram, 31
Eskalith, 21
Estazolam, 23
Eszopiclone, 29
Ethchlorvynol, 19
Ethinamate, 19
Euphoria, 59

F
Fastin, 123
Fenethylline, 124
Fenfluramine, 123
Fentanyl, 74
Fioricet, 17
Fiorinal, 17
Flunitrazepam, 22, 23
Fluoxetine, 31
Flurazepam, 23
Fluvoxamine, 31
Freebase, 112

G
GBL, 24, 25, 26, 27
GHB, 24, 25, 26, 27
Glutethimide, 19
Guarana, 123

H
Halazepam, 23
Halcion, 23
Haldol, 21
Haloperidol, 21
Hashish, 8
Hawaiian Woodrose, 48
Heroin, 76

Hycodan, 85
Hydrocodone, 84
Hydromorphone, 82
Hydroxyzine, 29
Hyperthermia, 183
Hypothermia, 183

I
Ice, 116
Imipramine, 31
Inapsine, 21
Inhalants, 62
Innovar, 75
Ionamin, 123
Isocarboxazide, 31

J
Jimson Weed, 44, 45

K
Kakuam, 99
Ketamine, 104, 105
Ketum, 99
Klonopin, 22, 23
Kratom, 98

L
Laughing Gas, 68
Lexapro, 31
Lexotan, 23
Librium, 23
Lithane, 21
Lithium, 20, 21
Lithobid, 21
Lofentanyl, 75
Lorazepam, 22, 23
Lorcet, 85
Lortab, 85
Loxapine, 21
Loxitane, 21
LSA, 48
LSD, 46
Ludiomil, 31
Luminal, 17
Lunesta, 29
Luvox, 31
Lysergic Acid Diethylamide, 46

M
Magic Mushrooms, 52
Maprotiline, 31
Marijuana, 2
Marplan, 31
Mazanor, 123
Mazindol, 123
MDMA, 34, 35
Mebaral, 17

Mellaril, 21
Meperidine, 86
Meperitab, 87
Mephobarbital, 17
Meprobamate, 19
Mescaline, 50, 51
Mesoridazine, 21
Metadate, 111
Metadol, 89
Methadone, 88
Methadose, 88
Methamphetamine, 111, 116
Methaqualone, 19
Methcathinone, 118
Methocarbamol, 19
Methohexital, 17
Methylphenidate, 111
Methyprylon, 19
Midazolam, 23
Miltown, 19
Mirtazapine, 31
Moban, 21
Modafinil, 124
Mogadan, 23
Molindone, 21
Moludar, 19
Morning Glory Seeds, 48
Morphine, 90
MS Contin, 91
Myristicin, 56

N
Nalbuphine, 97
Nardil, 31
Nefazodone, 31
Nimetazepam, 23
Niravam, 23
Nistenal, 123
Nitrazepam, 23
Nitrous Oxide, 68
Noctec, 19
Norpramine, 31
Nortriptyline, 31
Nubain, 97
Numbutal, 17
Nutmeg, 56

O
Olanzapine, 21
Opium, 92
Oxazepam, 23
Oxycocet, 95
Oxycodan, 95
Oxycodone, 94

OxyContin, 94, 95
Oxydose, 95
OxyFast, 95

P
Pamate, 31
Pamelor, 31
Papa Ecstasy, 34
Paral, 19
Paraldehyde, 19
Paraphernalia, 142
Paroxetine, 31
Paxil, 31
Paxipam, 23
PCP, 102
Pemoline, 111
Pentazocine, 97
Pentobarbital, 17
Pentothal, 17
Percocet, 94, 95
Perphenazine, 21
Peyote, 50, 51
Peyote Cactus, 51
Phenazepam, 23
Phencyclidine, 102
Phendimetrazine, 123
Phenelzine, 31
Phenergan, 21
Phenethylamines, 34
Phenmetrazine, 123
Phenobarbital, 17
Phentermine, 122, 123
Piperazines, 59
Placidyl, 19
Pliva, 29
Pondimin, 123
Prazepam, 23
Prelu-2, 123
Preludin, 123
Prochlorperazine, 21
Prolixin, 21
Promethazine, 21
Propoxyphene, 97
ProSom, 23
Protryptaline, 31
Provigil, 124
Prozac, 31
Pseudoephedrine, 123
Psilocin, 52
Psilocybin, 52

Q
Quaalude, 19
Quazepam, 23

Quetiapine Fumarate, 21

R
Redux, 123
Remeron, 31
Restoril, 23
Riphenidate, 111
Risperdal, 21
Risperidone, 21
Ritalin, 111
Rivotril, 22, 23
Robaxin, 19
Rofranil, 31
Rohypnol, 22, 23
roofies, 23
Roxanol, 91
Roxicet, 95

S
Salvia Divinorum, 54, 55
Sanorex, 123
Secobarbital, 17
Seconal, 17
Serax, 23
Serentil, 21
Seroquel, 21
Sertraline HCl, 31
Serzone, 31
Shulgin, Dr. Alex, 34
Sinequan, 31
Sinsemilla, 183
Slo-Phyllin, 124
Soma, 18, 19
Somnote, 19
Sonata, 28, 29
Special K, 104
Speed, 116
Stadol, 97
Starter Heroin, 80
Statistics, 166
Steroids, 125, 126
Sublimaze, 75
Subutex, 97
Sufenta, 75
Sufentanyl, 75
Supprettes, 19
Surmontil, 31
Synesthesia, 183

T
Tachycardia, 183
Talacen, 97
Talwin, 97
Taurine, 123
Temazepam, 23

TFMPP, 59
Thai Stick, 4
Thang, 99
Thiopental, 17
Thioridazine, 21
Thom, 99
Thorazine, 21
Tigan, 21
Tramadol, 97
Tranquilizers, 20
Tranylcypromine, 31
Tranzene, 23
Trazadone, 30, 31
Triazolam, 23
Trifluoromethylphenylpiperazine, 59
Trilafon, 21
Trimethobenzamide, 21
Trimipramine, 31
Triptil, 31
Tryptamines, 40, 41
Tuinal, 17
Tylox, 95

U
U4EUH, 59
Ultram, 97

V
Valium, 22, 23
Venlafaxine, 31
Versed, 23
Vicodin, 84
Vicoprofen, 85
Vistaral, 29
Vivactil, 31

W
Wellbutrin, 31

X
Xanax, 23
Xyrem, 24, 25, 26, 27

Y
Yohimbe, 123

Z
Zaleplon, 29
Zoloft, 31
Zolpidem, 29
Zyban, 31
Zyprexa, 21